Clinical Cases in Cardiology

Series editors:

Ravi V. Shah
Boston, MA, USA

Siddique A. Abbasi
Providence, RI, USA

James L. Januzzi
Boston, MA, USA

AF166651

Clinical cases are a key component in modern medical education, assisting the trainee or recertifying clinician to work through unusual cases using best practice techniques. Cardiology is a key discipline in this regard and is a highly visual subject requiring the reader to describe often very subtle differences in the presentation of patients and define accurately the diagnostic and management criteria on which to base their clinical decision-making.

This series of concise practical guides is designed to facilitate the clinical decision-making process by reviewing a number of cases and defining the various diagnostic and management decisions open to clinicians.

Each title will be illustrated and diverse in scope, enabling the reader to obtain relevant clinical information regarding both standard and unusual cases in a rapid, easy to digest format.

More information about this series at http://www.springer.com/series/14348

Atooshe Rohani

Clinical Cases in Cardio-Oncology

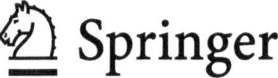

Atooshe Rohani
Northern Ontario School of Medicine
Thunder Bay, ON
Canada

ISSN 2523-3009   ISSN 2523-3017   (electronic)
Clinical Cases in Cardiology
ISBN 978-3-030-71154-2   ISBN 978-3-030-71155-9   (eBook)
https://doi.org/10.1007/978-3-030-71155-9

This Springer imprint is published by the registered company Springer
Nature Switzerland AG
The registered company address is: Gewerbestrasse 11, 6330 Cham, Switzerland

Clinical Cases in Cardio-Oncology is a great clinical reference for internists, cardiologists, and oncologists. I started practicing in the cardio-oncology field in beautiful Northwestern Ontario, Canada around 3 years ago. It was a new field for me and challenged me in many ways. I thoroughly enjoy practicing in this field and I hope by writing this book, I can share my expertise with my colleagues across the globe especially for early-career cardiologists and anyone wanting to start work in this very interesting field. I was inspired by and very appreciative of one of my first patients when I asked her for consent to share her clinical data in my book. She replied with an emphatic yes! She said she would do anything to help other cancer patients across the world. I remember on that day I felt so blessed to be her cardiologist on the challenging journey of breast cancer treatment. Gratefully I would find that all my patients were very willing to give consent to use their data. This book is because of them.

Contents

List of Abbreviations

ACEI	Angiotensin converting enzyme inhibitor
AF	Atrial fibrillation
AHA	American Heart Association
ARB	Angiotensin receptor blocker
ASCO	American Society of Clinical Oncology
ASE	American Society of echocardiography
AVRT	Atrioventricular reentrant tachycardia
BB	Beta-blocker
BMI	Body mass index
BNP	B-type natriuretic peptide
BPM	Beats per minute
CABG	Coronary artery bypass graft
CAD	Coronary artery disease
CCS class	Canadian Cardiovascular Society grading of angina pectoris
CHF	Congestive heart failure
CIED	Cardiovascular implantable electronic devices
CML	Chronic myelogenous leukemia
cMRI	Cardiac magnetic resonance imaging
CPAP	Continuous positive airway pressure
CRP	C-reactive protein
CTO	Chronic total occlusion

CVD	Cardiovascular disease
DCM	Dilated cardiomyopathy
DOAC	Direct oral anticoagulant
DVT	Deep vein thrombosis
FDA	Food and Drug Administration
FOLFIRI chemotherapy	FOL—folinic acid (leucovorin), F—fluorouracil (5-FU), IRI—irinotecan
FOLFOX	Folinic acid (leucovorin) "FOL", Fluorouracil (5-FU) "F", and Oxaliplatin (Eloxatin) "OX"
GI	Gastrointestinal
GLS	Global longitudinal strain
Gy	Gray
HF	Heart failure
HFmrEF	Heart failure with midrange ejection fraction
HFpEF	Heart failure with preserved ejection fraction
HFrEF	Heart failure with reduced ejection fraction
HTN	Hypertension
ICD	Implantable cardioverter-defibrillator
ICI	Immune checkpoint inhibitors
IMiD	Immunomodulatory drug
LAD	Left anterior descending artery
LCX	Left circumflex artery
LMWH	Low molecular weight heparin
LV	Left ventricle
LVEF	Left ventricular ejection fraction
MCA	Middle cerebral artery
mmol/L	Millimoles per litre
MUGA	Multigated acquisition
NSTEMI	Non-ST-elevation myocardial infarction
NT-proBNP	N-terminal pro–B-type natriuretic peptide

NYHA	New York Heart Association
PAH	Pulmonary arterial hypertension
PASP	Pulmonary artery systolic pressure
PCI	Percutaneous Coronary Intervention
PE	Pulmonary embolism
PPM	Permanent pacemaker
RCA	Right coronary artery
RVOT	Right ventricular outflow
TEE	Transesophageal echocardiogram
TGCC	Testicular germ-cell cancer
TKI	Tyrosine Kinase Inhibitors
TRV	Tricuspid regurgitant jet velocity
TTE	Transthoracic echocardiogram
TEE	Trans esophageal echocardiography
VEGF	Vascular endothelial growth factor
VKA	Vitamin K antagonist
VTE	Venous thromboembolism

Chapter 1
Introduction

My book Clinical Cardio-Oncology Cases, has 25 chapters which I can confidently say addresses most of the common clinical scenarios in a cardio-oncology clinic from dealing with anthracycline and 5 FU cardiotoxicities, myocarditis by immune checkpoint inhibitors, Dasatinib pulmonary toxicities to rare side effects from newer generations of cancer treatment and some general topics like as long QT interval, atrial fibrillation and Deep Vein Thrombosis in cancer patients.

Every chapter include abstract, description of a clinical case, (history, physical examination, investigations and plan of treatment) followed by clinical pearls about diagnostic approach and treatment options based on the latest guidelines.

I think internist, cardiologists and oncologists, with interest in cardio oncology will benefit the most from this book.

Obviously, it is not a textbook in cardio oncology, but it is a fantastic practical bedside guide.

I wish you will enjoy reading it as much as I enjoyed writing it.

Almost 20 years ago, I chose cardiology as my specialty in medicine because I am passionate about caring for people with all my heart. I was offered an opportunity to work in the field of cardio-oncology about 3 years ago.

© The Author(s), under exclusive license to Springer Nature Switzerland AG 2021
A. Rohani, *Clinical Cases in Cardio-Oncology*, Clinical Cases in Cardiology, https://doi.org/10.1007/978-3-030-71155-9_1

As an empath, I always believed that from an emotional standpoint, it would be challenging to be involved in the care of cancer patients. Cardio-oncology has forced me to step out of my comfort zone and in doing so, I have found another passion in medicine.

I have received support for the writing of this book from my dear friend, Carolyn Leonzio. I would like to thank her for this and for her unconditional love and friendship on my journey.

I would also like to take the opportunity to thank all my patients for giving me the opportunity to be involved in their care. It has been a pleasure in helping them maintain a healthy heart while enduring their very challenging journey of cancer treatments. I appreciate all kind referrals from oncologists in Thunder Bay Regional health sciences to cardio-oncology clinic.

Also, I wish to express my gratitude to Dr. Zaki Ahmed, the chief of staff of Thunder Bay Regional Health Sciences Centre for all his supports during the writing of this book.

Furthermore, I am always feeling so lucky to have a great family and friends, definetely without their help, writing of this book was impossible.

Finally, I want to dedicate this book to the light and love of my life, my lovely genius daughter, Parmida.

Out beyond ideas of wrongdoing and rightdoing, there is a field. I'll meet you there.
Rumi

Chapter 2
Dasatinib Induced Pleural Effusion and Pulmonary Hypertension

Clinical Case

Patient was a 65 years old female with BCR-ABL-positive chronic myelogenous leukemia (CML). She has been receiving Dasatinib 70 mg twice daily with excellent response with 4.4 log reduction on the latest molecular study for around 10 months.

She presented with gradually worsening shortness of breath and NYHA class 2–3. On examination she has stable vital signs but decreased air entry to the 2/3 of right side of her chest.

She underwent a chest X ray which confirmed moderate to large size right side pleural effusion (Fig. 2.1). Thoracentesis showed: exudative effusion with lymphocyte predominant.

Echocardiogram revealed normal left ventricular wall motion and systolic function and no significant valvular abnormalities.

Dose of Dasatinib reduced from 70 mg twice daily to 100 mg daily. She was started on daily Lasix 20 mg. Eventually dose of dasatinib reduced to 50 mg daily due to recurrent pleural effusions. Then, Dasatinib discontinued due to proteinuria and imatinib 400 mg/day started.

© The Author(s), under exclusive license to Springer Nature Switzerland AG 2021
A. Rohani, *Clinical Cases in Cardio-Oncology*, Clinical Cases in Cardiology, https://doi.org/10.1007/978-3-030-71155-9_2

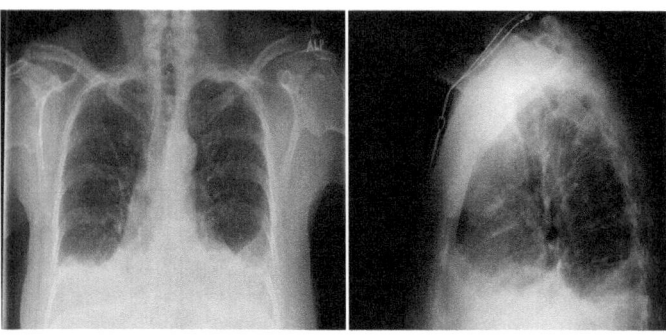

FIGURE 2.1 Bilateral pleural effusion on chest X ray

Imatinib was also stopped due to grade 3 heart failure, periorbital edema, increased shortness of breath and nonproductive cough.

Finally, she was started on bosutinib 400 mg three times per day. Two months later, she again presented with large left side pleural effusion (Fig. 2.2). Thoracentesis performed, which showed lymphocytic predominant exudates. Dose of bosutinib reduced to 400 mg daily. On follow up, there was no recurrence of pleural effusion.

Clinical Pearls

1. Dasatinib is used for treatment of BCR-ABL-positive chronic myeloid leukemia and Philadelphia chromosome-positive acute lymphoblastic leukemia.
2. Dasatinib is associated with QT prolongation: Moderate risk (5–10% incidence) Close monitoring of potassium and magnesium, avoidance of drugs that can prolong the QTc interval should be considered [1–3].
3. Dasatinib could cause pleural effusion among 29% of patients, this decrease to 1–10% for bosutinib. Pleural effusion is mostly bilateral and has exudative pattern [4, 5].

    (a) Pleural effusion interestingly could be associated with better clinical leukemia response to dasatinib [4].

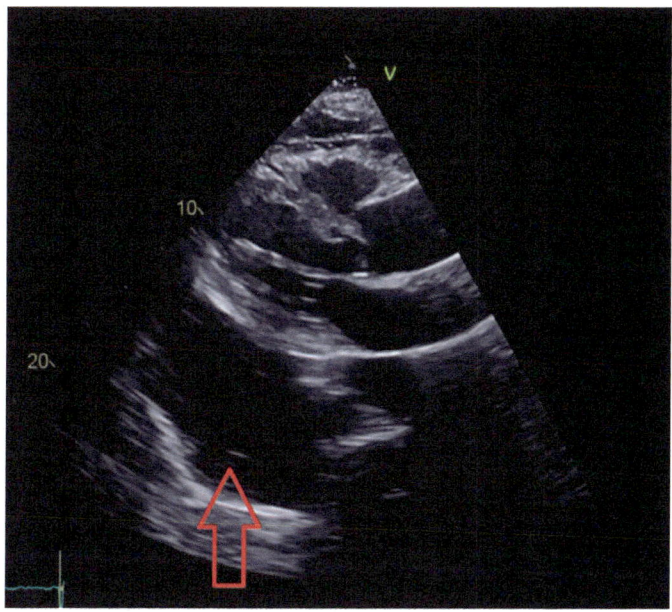

FIGURE 2.2 TTE, para sternal view: red arrow shows left side pleural effusion recurrence after starting patient on bosutinib

(b) Risk factors for development of pleural effusions [5, 6]:

- Twice daily dosing of dasatinib
- Older age
- Lymphocytosis
- Prior cardiac history
- Autoimmune disease

(c) Optimal treatment of pleural effusion is not known: no treatment is necessary for asymptomatic and small effusions. For larger, symptomatic effusion combinations or one of the following therapies could be considered [6]:

- Altering the dose of dasatinib from 70 mg twice daily to 100 mg daily.
- Systemic glucocorticoids.
- Diuretics.

- Thoracentesis.
- Dasatinib/bosutinib interruption or discontinuation.
- Pleurodesis.

4. Reversible Pulmonary arterial hypertension (PAH) is another adverse side effect of Dasatinib treatment, and usually occurs after 8–48 months of treatment.

   (a) PAH should be suspected in patients with fatigue, peripheral edema tachypnea, and progressive or unexplained shortness of breath.
   (b) Transthoracic echocardiography (TTE) should be considered as the initial modality of choice for estimation of pulmonary artery systolic pressure (PASP) [6]:

      - If tricuspid regurgitant jet velocity (TRV) is >3.4 m s^{-1}, probability of PAH is high (Fig. 2.3)
      - If TRV is ≤2.8 m s^{-1}, probability of PH is low.

   (c) When TRV is between 2.9 and 3.4 m s^{-1} for diagnosis of PAH, other echocardiographic features of PAH must be present:

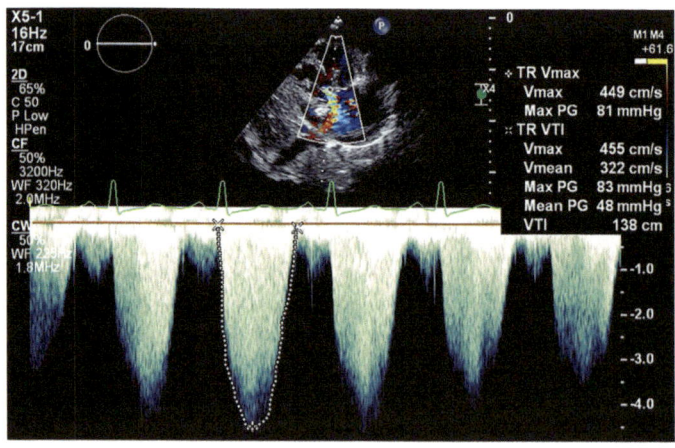

FIGURE 2.3 TRV = 4.49 m s^{-1} >3.8, and peak pressure gradient of 83 mmHg in favor of severe PAH. Doppler echo of TV

- Right ventricular outflow Doppler acceleration time <105 ms
- Mid-systolic notching of right ventricular outflow (RVOT) pulse wave Doppler, (Fig. 2.4)
- D shape septum (flattening of the interventricular septum): Fig. 2.5
- Dilated inferior vena cava (IVC).

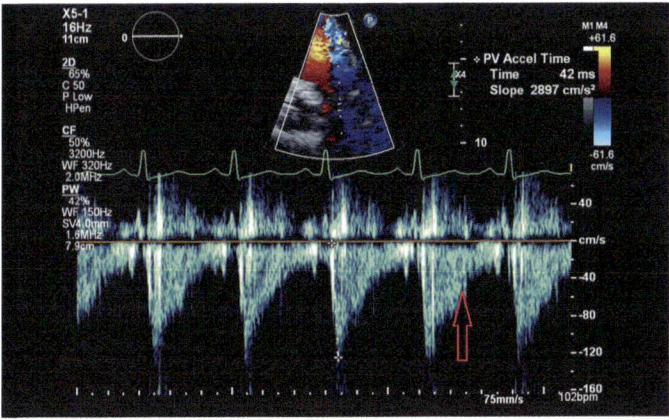

FIGURE 2.4 Mid-systolic notch on the pulmonary artery Doppler flow tracing (red arrow). Right ventricular outflow Doppler acceleration time <105 ms in this picture, it is 42 ms

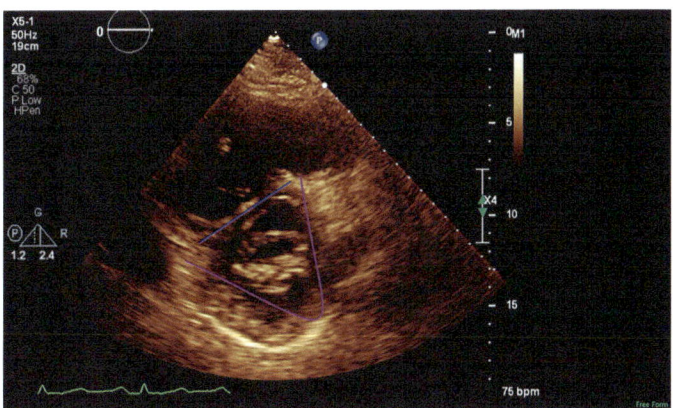

FIGURE 2.5 D shape septum in systole, consistent with RV pressure overload

(d) Re-challenge should be avoided in dasatinib-induced PAH [6].

(e) After stopping dasatinib, PAH is usually reversible.

(f) DASISION trial supported 100 mg daily dose of dasatinib as a safe therapy for treatment of CML with 28% incidence of pleural effusion mostly in the first year after treatment with Dasatinib [7–9].

(g) Lung toxicities with other anticancer drugs (bleomycin, gemcitabine, oxaliplatin, bortezomib, cytarabine, anthracyclines and lenalidomide) has been observed.

(h) Bleomycin lung toxicity is related to the cumulative dose and is more common in patients with impaired renal function and age more than 40 years old; Idiosyncratic reactions with other agents has been observed [10–13].

References

1. Goldblatt M, Huggins JT, Doelken P, Gurung P, Sahn SA. Dasatinib-induced pleural effusions: a lymphatic network disorder? Am J Med Sci. 2009;338:414–7.

2. Huang YM, Wang CH, Huang JS, Yeh KY, Lai CH, Wu TH, et al. Dasatinib-related chylothorax. Turk J Haematol. 2015;32:68–72.

3. aydas S. Dasatinib, large granular lymphocytosis, and pleural effusion: useful or adverse effect? Crit Rev Oncol Hematol. 2014;89:242–7.

4. Montani D, Bergot E, Günther S, et al. Pulmonary arterial hypertension in patients treated by dasatinib. Circulation. 2012;125(17):2128–37.

5. Moguillansky NI, Fakih HAM, Wingard JR. Bosutinib induced pleural effusions: Case report and review of tyrosine kinase inhibitors induced pulmonary toxicity. Respir Med Case Rep. 2017;21:154–7. https://doi.org/10.1016/j.rmcr.2017.05.003. PMID: 28560147; PMCID: PMC5435591

6. 2015 ESC/ERS Guidelines for the diagnosis and treatment of pulmonary hypertension: The Joint Task Force for the Diagnosis and Treatment of Pulmonary Hypertension of the European Society of Cardiology (ESC) and the European Respiratory Society (ERS) Endorsed by: Association for European Paediatric

and Congenital Cardiology (AEPC), International Society for Heart and Lung Transplantation (ISHLT).

7. Orlandi EM, Rocca B, Pazzano AS, Ghio S. Reversible pulmonary arterial hypertension likely related to long-term, low dose dasatinib treatment for chronic myeloid leukaemia. Leuk Res. 2012;36(1):e4–6.

8. Cortes JE, Saglio G, Kantarjian HM, et al. Final 5-year study results of DASISION: the dasatinib versus imatinib study in treatment-naïve chronic myeloid leukemia patients trial. J Clin Oncol. 2016;34(20):2333–40.

9. Caldemeyer L, Dugan M, Edwards J, Akard L. Long-term side effects of tyrosine kinase inhibitors in chronic myeloid leukemia. Curr Hematol Malign Rep. 2016;11(2):71–9.

10. Sleijfer S. Bleomycin-induced pneumonitis. Chest. 2001;120(2):617–24. https://doi.org/10.1378/chest.120.2.617. PMID: 11502668.

11. O'Sullivan JM, Huddart RA, Norman AR, Nicholls J, Dearnaley DP, Horwich A. Predicting the risk of bleomycin lung toxicity in patients with germ-cell tumours. Ann Oncol. 2003;14(1):91–6. https://doi.org/10.1093/annonc/mdg020. PMID: 12488299.

12. Jacobs C, Slade M, Lavery B. Doxorubicin and BOOP. A possible near fatal association. Clin Oncol (R Coll Radiol). 2002;14(3):262. https://doi.org/10.1053/clon.2002.0071. PMID: 12109837.

13. Miyakoshi S, Kami M, Yuji K, Matsumura T, Takatoku M, Sasaki M, Narimatsu H, Fujii T, Kawabata M, Taniguchi S, Ozawa K, Oshimi K. Severe pulmonary complications in Japanese patients after bortezomib treatment for refractory multiple myeloma. Blood. 2006;107(9):3492–4. https://doi.org/10.1182/blood-2005-11-4541. Epub 2006 Jan 12. PMID: 16410442.

Chapter 3
Ponatinib Induced Stroke

Clinical Case

A 65-year-old male patient with BCR-ABL1 T315I-positive CML in chronic phase, resistant to dasatinib and nilotinib treatment, was started on the third generation of TKI: ponatinib (45 mg once daily) prior to allogeneic stem cell transplant.

He has background history of hyperlipidemia, and there was no history of cardiovascular disease.

Within 2 weeks of initiation of therapy, he developed left sided hemiplegia, slurred speech and hemiparesis. He was diagnosed with Middle cerebral artery (MCA) stroke. Ponatinib was immediately stopped and brain CT scan revealed the hyperdense MCA sign. 24 hours Holter monitoring showed no episode of Atrial fibrillation. Echocardiogram revealed Normal LV size and function with No significant valvular abnormalities or source of embolism. CT angiography of carotid arteries showed mild stenosis, but less than 50% of both internal carotid arteries. Therefore, it was concluded that stroke was ponatinib-induced thrombosis in middle cerebral artery. He received intravenous alteplase and underwent Mechanical thrombectomy. He did require extensive Neurology Rehabilitation including Physiotherapy and Occupational Therapy. He was gradually improved.

© The Author(s), under exclusive license to Springer Nature Switzerland AG 2021
A. Rohani, *Clinical Cases in Cardio-Oncology*, Clinical Cases in Cardiology, https://doi.org/10.1007/978-3-030-71155-9_3

Clinical Pearls [1–7]

1. Embolic events, venous and arterial and thromboses occur in more than 27% of patients receiving Ponatinib treatment.
2. Vascular complications are not dose dependent, but many hematologists decrease the dose to the lowest effective dose.
3. Albeit there are no prospective data, there is a recommendation from many clinicians to provide aspirin to patients on ponatinib treatment especially those who are more than 60 years old.
4. Aggressive management of cardiovascular risk factors (hypertension, hyperlipidemia, diabetes, smoking) is strongly recommended. Emergent high blood pressure reported in over two-thirds of patients who treated with ponatinib; Blood pressure needs to be monitored closely. Ponatinib must stopped if there is resistant hypertension. Evaluation for renal artery stenosis should be considered in case of worsening or resistant hypertension [7].
5. Patients taking ponatinib should be monitored closely for signs and symptoms of left ventricular systolic dysfunction, as 4% of patients on ponatinib treatment have developed left ventricular systolic dysfunction, which could be quite serious with fatalities. Ponatinib therapy should be stopped if new or worsening heart failure occurs.
6. Patient's education about stroke, venous thromboembolism and heart failure symptoms are very important.
7. Arrythmia in the form of both symptomatic brady arrhythmias, Fig. 3.1 (1%), and supraventricular tachyarrhythmias

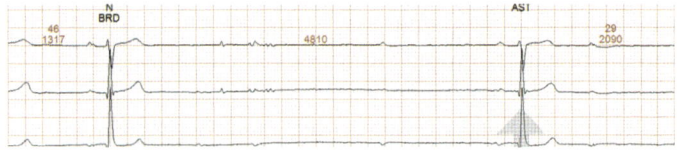

FIGURE 3.1 Bradyarrhythmia, advanced AV block

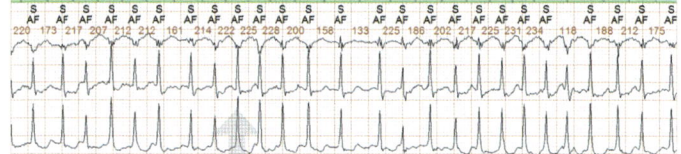

FIGURE 3.2 Atrial fibrillation with rapid ventricular response

(predominantly atrial fibrillation, Fig. 3.2) is also noted in around 5% of patients on Ponatinib treatment.

References

1. Gambacorti-Passerini C, Piazza R. Choosing the right TKI for chronic myeloid leukemia: when the truth lies in "long-term" safety and efficacy. Am J Hematol. 2011;86(7):531–2. https://doi.org/10.1002/ajh.22084.
2. Dahlén T, Edgren G, Lambe M, et al. Cardiovascular events associated with use of tyrosine kinase inhibitors in chronic myeloid leukemia: a population-based cohort study. Ann Intern Med. 2016;165:161.
3. Cortes JE, Kim DW, Pinilla-Ibarz J, leCoutre P, Paquette R, Chuah C, Nicolini FE, Apperley JF. A phase 2 trial of ponatinib in Philadelphia chromosome-positive leukemias. N Engl J Med. 2013;369:1.
4. Totzeck M, Mincu RI, Mrotzek S, Schadendorf D, Rassaf T. Cardiovascular diseases in patients receiving small molecules with anti-vascular endothelial growth factor activity: a meta-analysis of approximately 29,000 cancer patients. Eur J Prev Cardiol. 2018;25(5):482–94.
5. Massaro F, Molica M, Breccia M. Ponatinib: a review of efficacy and safety. Curr Cancer Drug Targets. 2018;18(9):847–56.
6. Singh AP, Glennon MS, Umbarkar P, et al. Ponatinib-induced cardiotoxicity: delineating the signalling mechanisms and potential rescue strategies. Cardiovasc Res. 2019;115(5):966–77.
7. Santoro M, Accurso V, Mancuso S, et al. Management of ponatinib in patients with chronic myeloid leukemia with cardiovascular risk factors. Chemotherapy. 2019;64(4):205–9.

Chapter 4
Nilotinib Induced Peripheral Artery Occlusive Disease

Clinical Case

Patient was a 62-year-old male with Philadelphia chromosome–positive CML started on nilotinib. His cardiovascular risk factors include hypertension and hyperlipidemia.

He had no previous history of cardiovascular disease.

After 1 year of Nilotinib treatment, he presented with thigh pain brought by activity and relieved with rest (intermittent claudication). On examination he had dry, shiny, and hairless skin on his left lower extremity with a dusky flush spreading proximally from the toes in the dependent position. Popliteal pulse was not palpable on left side. Bedside Doppler Ultrasound showed ankle brachial index of 0.8 on left side. Risk factors modification and supervised exercise therapy started. He was referred to vascular surgeon and started on 81 mg of aspirin. He underwent CT angiogram of both lower extremities which showed left long-segment Trans-Atlantic Inter-Society (TASC) II D femoropopliteal occlusive disease. He underwent bypass surgery. After this, Nilotinib was stopped and switched to dasatinib 100 mg p.o. daily.

There was no recurrence of his symptoms in 1 year follow up.

© The Author(s), under exclusive license to Springer Nature Switzerland AG 2021
A. Rohani, *Clinical Cases in Cardio-Oncology*, Clinical Cases in Cardiology, https://doi.org/10.1007/978-3-030-71155-9_4

Clinical Pearls [1–5]

1. Aggressive cardiovascular risk factor modification is essential in patients on nilotinib treatment.
2. Nilotinib associated with QT prolongation, (Low risk: 1–5% incidence). Hypokalemia and hypomagnesemia should be promptly corrected. Avoidance of CYP3A4 inhibitors and medications that may prolong the QTc interval suggested [4].
3. Pericardial, Pleural effusions, ascites, and pulmonary edema, sometimes in severe form has also been reported with Nilotinib treatment.

References

1. Quintás-Cardama A, Kantarjian H, Cortes J. Nilotinib-associated vascular events. Clin Lymphoma Myeloma Leuk. 2012;12(5):337–340.2012.04.005.
2. Tefferi A, Letendre L. Nilotinib treatment-associated peripheral artery disease and sudden death: yet another reason to stick to imatinib as front-line therapy for chronic myelogenous leukemia. Am J Hematol. 2011;86(7):610–1. https://doi.org/10.1002/ajh.22051.
3. Aichberger KJ, Herndlhofer S, Schernthaner GH, et al. Progressive peripheral arterial occlusive disease and other vascular events during nilotinib therapy in CML. Am J Hematol. 2011;86(7):533–9. https://doi.org/10.1002/ajh.22037.
4. Porta-Sánchez A, Gilbert C, Spears D, et al. Incidence, diagnosis, and management of QT prolongation induced by cancer therapies: a systematic review. J Am Heart Assoc. 2017;6(12)
5. Norgren L, Hiatt WR, Dormandy JA, et al. Inter-society consensus for the management of peripheral arterial disease (TASC II). J Vasc Surg. 2007;45 Suppl:S5–S67.

Chapter 5
Imatinib Cardiotoxicity

Clinical Case

Patient was a 65-year-old female presented to the emergency department with an episode of palpitation lasted for half an hour, peripheral edema, shortness of breath and mild increase in troponin. She had history of palpitation for many years. She had five episodes of palpitation, lasted for around 5–10 min over the month before this presentation. These episodes spontaneously terminated with no need to seek medical attention. She was known for CML on imatinib treatment. She also had obstructive sleep apnea on Continuous positive airway pressure (CPAP).

On examination, blood pressure 133/82 mmHg, pulse rate of 160 beats per minute, regular, temperature 36.7, oxygen saturation 95% on room air. Chest was clear. Heart had normal S1, S2, with no murmur. There was peripheral edema 1+ below the knee. Pedal pulses were palpable.

She converted to normal sinus rhythm with 12 mg of IntraVenous adenosine.

She had normal level of thyroid-stimulating hormone (TSH).

© The Author(s), under exclusive license to Springer Nature Switzerland AG 2021
A. Rohani, *Clinical Cases in Cardio-Oncology*, Clinical Cases in Cardiology, https://doi.org/10.1007/978-3-030-71155-9_5

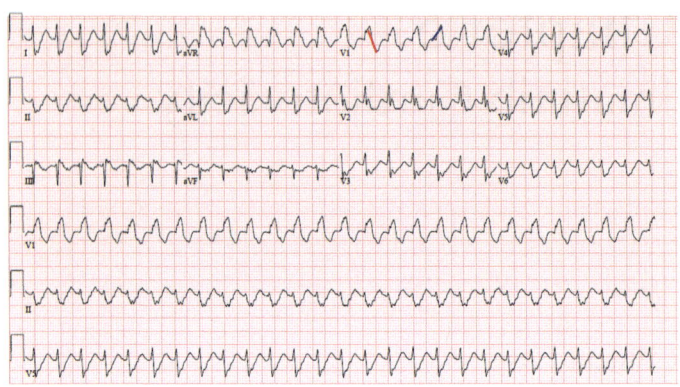

FIGURE 5.1 Narrow complex tachycardia with heart rate of 160 bpm, RP (red) interval more than PR (blue) interval

Chest CT scan showed no evidence of pulmonary embolism.

Her baseline ECG was normal sinus rhythm, bi-fascicular block (right bundle branch block and left anterior fascicular block) with heart rate of 75 beats per minute. Her ECG on presentation to the hospital showed regular tachycardia with heart rate of 160 bpm, RP interval more than PR interval (Fig. 5.1).

Echocardiogram showed LV ejection fraction of 45% with basal inferior and basal inferoseptal wall hypokinesia.

Coronary angiogram revealed chronic total occlusion (CTO) of right coronary artery (RCA) and Left to right collaterals from LAD septal perforators (Fig. 5.2). Patient was started on stepwise combination of three agents: ACE inhibitor, beta-blocker and Diuretic for treatment of HFmrEF. He also underwent successful Atrioventricular reentrant tachycardia (AVRT), left lateral accessory pathway ablation. It was difficult to conclude these cardiovascular complications was drug related or a process of aging and diffuse atherosclerosis, however imatinib could exacerbate underlying cardiovascular disease in this patient.

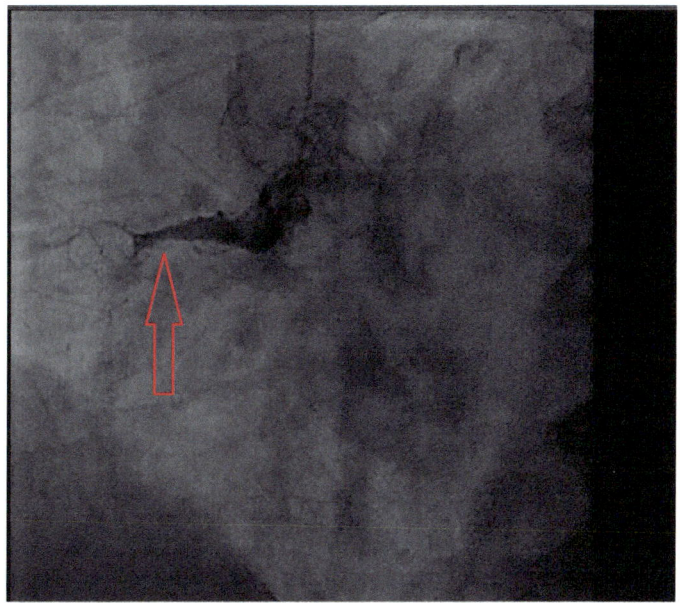

FIGURE 5.2 CTO of RCA, red arrow on coronary angiogram

Clinical Pearls [1–6]

- Advanced age and other comorbidities increase risk of cardiotoxicity with imatinib. Overall rate of imatinib-related cardiac toxicity is between 0.7 and 1.3%.
- Heart failure, peripheral and periorbital edema, ischemia/infarction, hypertension, and hypotension are reported side effects of imatinib treatment.
- Patients with hypereosinophilic syndrome and cardiac involvement or patients with chronic eosinophilic leukemia/myelodysplastic/myeloproliferative (MDS/MPD) disease associated with high eosinophil levels might present with cardiogenic shock with initiation of imatinib treatment, which is reversible with systemic steroids, and temporary holding of imatinib. These subgroups of patients

might benefit from monitoring by echocardiogram, serum troponin and prophylactic systemic steroids (for 1–2 weeks) with the initiation of imatinib.

- Heart failure is a well-known side effect of imatinib, and patients should be informed and monitored carefully for symptoms and signs of heart failure, however there is no need for obtaining a baseline echocardiogram prior to starting imatinib.
- Pericardial effusion and atrial fibrillation are also rare side effects of imatinib.
- Patients must be notified about the rare but serious adverse event of heart failure with imatinib treatment as part of informed consent.

References

1. Verweij J, Casali PG, Kotasek D, et al. Imatinib does not induce cardiac left ventricular failure in gastrointestinal stromal tumours patients: analysis of EORTC-ISG-AGITG study 62005. Eur J Cancer. 2007;43(6):974–8.
2. Atallah E, Durand JB, Kantarjian H, Cortes J. Congestive heart failure is a rare event in patients receiving imatinib therapy. Blood. 2007;110(4):1233–7.
3. Guilhot F. Indications for imatinib mesylate therapy and clinical management. Oncologist. 2004;9(3):271–81.
4. Kerkelä R, Grazette L, Yacobi R, et al. Cardiotoxicity of the cancer therapeutic agent imatinib mesylate. Nat Med. 2006;12(8):908–16.
5. Hatfield A, Owen S, Pilot PR. In reply to 'Cardiotoxicity of the cancer therapeutic agent imatinib mesylate'. Nat Med. 2007;13(1):13. Author reply 15-6. PMID: 17206118. https://doi.org/10.1038/nm0107-13a.
6. Mann DL. Targeted cancer therapeutics: the heartbreak of success. Nat Med. 2006;12(8):881–2. https://doi.org/10.1038/nm0806-881. PMID: 16892027.

Chapter 6
Doxorubicin Induced Heart Failure with Reduced Ejection Fraction

Clinical Case

Patient was a 62 years old woman with invasive ductal carcinoma of the right breast, treated with lumpectomy, chemotherapy with doxorubicin, (375 mg of doxorubicin per body surface area) cyclophosphamide and Taxol, 3 years prior to this presentation. She presented this time with exertional shortness of breath, NYHA class II to the hospital. She also had on and off chest pain with severity scale of 2/10. It was not exertional in nature with no obvious alleviating or aggravating factor.

Physical examination revealed elevated JVP, bibasilar crackles and 2+ peripheral edema. Electrocardiogram showed normal sinus rhythm with occasional PVCs (right bundle and inferior axis configuration).

Echocardiogram revealed severely enlarged left ventricle (Fig. 6.1) and ejection fraction of 15% by 3D. She had normal coronary angiogram. She was diagnosed with dilated cardiomyopathy, secondary to doxorubicin cardiotoxicity. Unfortunately, no echocardiogram was available over the 3 years course of chemo/radiotherapy.

© The Author(s), under exclusive license to Springer Nature Switzerland AG 2021
A. Rohani, *Clinical Cases in Cardio-Oncology*, Clinical Cases in Cardiology, https://doi.org/10.1007/978-3-030-71155-9_6

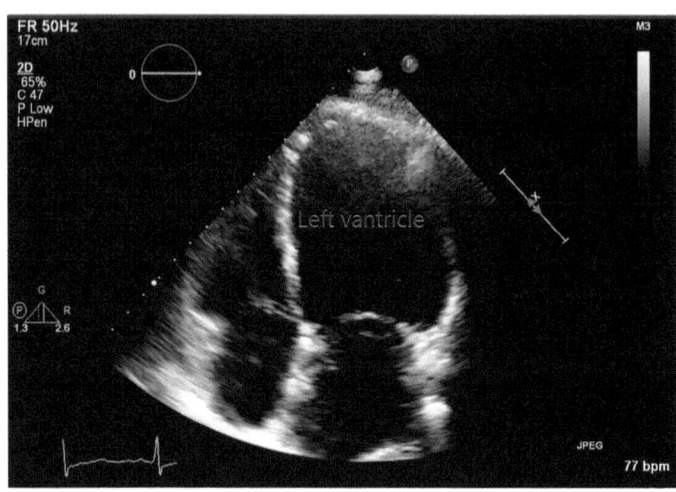

FIGURE 6.1 Enlarged left ventricle with poor systolic function, apical four chamber view in TTE

She was started on guideline-directed medical therapy and after 3 months her LV EF increased to 32%, still in NYHA class 2. Ramipril then switched to Sacubitril/valsartan (Entresto) and she underwent ICD insertion for primary prevention.

On 2 years follow up, she was stable and euvolemic however still with LVEF of 34%. Unfortunately, again she was diagnosed with biopsy-proven invasive ductal carcinoma of right breast and this time she underwent modified radical mastectomy.

Clinical Pearls [1–10]

Risk Factors for Developing Cardiotoxicity with Anthracycline

- Older age (>65 years) or young age (<4 years old)
- Female gender.
- Preexisting cardiovascular disease.

TABLE 6.1 Different anthracycline chemotherapy and incidence of left ventricular dysfunction

Doxorubicin (Adriamycin)	Incidence of LV dysfunction
400 mg/m^2	3–5%
550 mg/m^2	7–26%
700 mg/m^2	18–48%
Idarubicin (>90 mg/m^2)	5–18%
Epirubicin (>900 mg/m^2)	0.9–11.4%

- Presence of ≥2 cardiovascular risk factors including hypertension, smoking, hyperlipidemia, obesity, diabetes.
- High cumulative dose of anthracycline exposure. (Table 6.1 summarizes relationship between dose of different anthracyclines and incidence of left ventricular dysfunction.)
- Radiation therapy and concomitant use of trastuzumab.
- There is a recent study published by Dr. Abdel-Qadir et al., they developed a prediction model for major adverse cardiovascular events after early stage breast cancer: They considered past medical history of heart failure as the highest score among other risk factors (hypertension, diabetes, atrial fibrillation, peripheral arterial disease, chronic kidney disease, cerebrovascular disease, chronic obstructive pulmonary disease and ischemic heart disease.)There is an increment score for increase in age more than 40 years old, for example age more than 80 years old will add 31 scores to this prediction model [10].
- This risk score estimates cardiovascular prognosis and is useful to discuss the risk of cardiotoxic treatment with the patient and oncologist.
- A risk-benefit analysis of available treatment options should be performed before starting patient on anthracycline chemotherapy, careful monitoring of LVEF preferably by 3D echocardiography suggested; multigated acquisition (MUGA) or cardiac MRI (CMR) could be considered if echo is technically difficult or result is indecisive or inconsistent.

Arrythmia and anthracyclines

- Most arrhythmias occur with anthracyclines is secondary to cardiomyopathy, however ventricular arrhythmias can happen during administration or the early phase of chemotherapy.
- During the first cycle of therapy, arrhythmias reported in ≤65.5% of patients [12].
- ECG changes is not dose dependent.
- QTc interval prolongation seen with anthracyclines.
- AF has been reported with 10.3% incidence in one study [13].
- As Amiodarone is a P-glycoprotein/ATP-binding cassette sub-family B member 1 (ABCB1) Inhibitor, it increases serum concentration of Doxorubicin and this combination should be avoided.

Definition of Cardiotoxicity

LVEF <50% or decrease in LVEF of >10 percentage points from baseline.

Incidence:
Cardiotoxicity seen among 9% of patients receiving chemotherapy with Doxorubicin.

Time course:
The average onset of cardiotoxicity after completion of chemotherapy is 3.5 months, however 98% of cardiotoxicity was observed within the first year.

Late presentation occurs predominantly within 2–3 years of anthracycline exposure, the latest reported presentation was around 30 years after exposure.

Diagnosis

Anthracycline cardiotoxicity is a diagnosis of exclusion after other causes of HF (heart failure) or LV systolic dysfunction is ruled out.

- Exclusion of coronary artery disease and valvular heart disease is very important.
- In patients with leukemia, exclusion of endotoxemic shock from gram-negative infection and differentiation syndrome associated with ATRA and arsenic trioxide should be considered as differential diagnosis of heart failure with reduced ejection fraction.
- Subclinical cardiomyopathy is defined by American Society of echocardiography (ASE) by a 15% drop in global longitudinal strain (GLS). There is limited data if any treatment intervention could prevent further deterioration of LV systolic function.

Frequency of Echocardiogram

- In asymptomatic patients, if cumulative doxorubicin dose is less than 240 mg/m^2: one echocardiogram should be done at the baseline, another one at the completion of therapy, and last one at 6 months after completion of treatment should be considered.
- If doxorubicin dose exceeds 240 mg/m^2, evaluation is performed at 240 mg/m^2 and after each additional 50 mg/m^2 of doxorubicin.
- In patients with symptoms or signs of HF, echocardiogram should be repeated as soon as possible.

Prevention

- Close monitoring of blood pressure in hypertensive patients and optimizing of cardiac risk factors should be considered in all patients.
- Dexrazoxane: is FDA-approved drug for prevention of anthracycline cardiomyopathy in patients with metastatic breast cancer when lifetime dose of anthracycline exceeds 300 mg/m^2.
- American Heart Association endorses cardiovascular benefits of structured exercise to cancer patients.

Cardioprotective Strategy

1. Combination of an ACE inhibitor with carvedilol or nebivolol should be considered for all patients with LVEF >40 and <50% and no current or past HF.
2. Standard guideline-directed medical therapy for Heart Failure (GDMT) should be promptly started when diagnosis of heart failure with reduced ejection fraction is made.

   - The total lifetime dose of doxorubicin should be limited to 450 mg/m^2.
   - Infusional regimen and liposomal formulation of anthracyclines could reduce risk of cardiotoxicity.
   - Decline in LVEF to under 40%, or a 15 absolute percentage points to <50% prompts holding anthracyclines and utilizing a non-anthracycline-based regimen.

References

1. Cardinale D, Colombo A, Bacchiani G, Tedeschi I, Meroni CA, Veglia F, et al. Early detection of anthracycline cardiotoxicity and improvement with heart failure therapy. Circulation. 2015;131(22):1981–8.
2. Vejpongsa P, Yeh ET. Prevention of anthracycline-induced cardiotoxicity: challenges and opportunities. J Am Coll Cardiol. 2014;64(9):938–45.
3. McGowan JV, Chung R, Maulik A, Piotrowska I, Walker JM, Yellon DM. Anthracycline chemotherapy and cardiotoxicity. Cardiovasc Drugs Ther. 2017;31(1):63–75.
4. ipshultz SE, Alvarez JA, Scully RE. Anthracycline associated cardiotoxicity in survivors of childhood cancer. Heart. 2008;94(4):525–33.
5. Reichardt P, Tabone MD, Mora J, Morland B, Jones RL. Risk-benefit of dexrazoxane for preventing anthracycline-related cardiotoxicity: re-evaluating the European labeling. Future Oncol. 2018;14(25):2663–76.
6. Lipshultz SE. Letter by Lipshultz regarding article, "anthracycline cardiotoxicity: worrisome enough to have you quaking?". Circ Res. 2018;122(7):e62–3.

7. Lipshultz SE, Herman EH. Anthracycline cardiotoxicity: the importance of horizontally integrating pre-clinical and clinical research. Cardiovasc Res. 2018;114(2):205–9.

8. Choi HS, Park ES, Kang HJ, Shin HY, Noh CI, Yun YS, et al. Dexrazoxane for preventing anthracycline cardiotoxicity in children with solid tumors. J Korean Med Sci. 2010;25(9):1336–42.

9. Ganatra S, Nohria A, Shah S, Groarke JD, Sharma A, Venesy D, et al. Upfront dexrazoxane for the reduction of anthracycline-induced cardiotoxicity in adults with preexisting cardiomyopathy and cancer: a consecutive case series. Cardio-Oncology. 2019;5(1):1.

10. Abdel-Qadir H, Thavendiranathan P, Austin PC, Lee DS, Amir E, Tu JV, et al. Development and validation of a multivariable prediction model for major adverse cardiovascular events after early stage breast cancer: a population-based cohort study. Eur Heart J. 2019;40(48):3913–20.

11. Ryberg M, Nielsen D, Cortese G, Nielsen G, Skovsgaard T, Andersen PK. New insight into epirubicin cardiac toxicity: competing risks analysis of 1097breast cancer patients. J Natl Cancer Inst. 2008;100:1058–67.

12. Yeh ET, Bickford CL. Cardiovascular complications of cancer therapy: incidence, pathogenesis, diagnosis, and management. J Am Coll Cardiol. 2009;53:2231–47.

13. Kilickap S, Barista I, Akgul E, Aytemir K, Aksoy S, Tekuzman G. Early and late arrhythmogenic effects of doxorubicin. South Med J. 2007;100:262–5.

Chapter 7
Trastuzumab-Related Cardiotoxicity

Clinical Case

Patient was a 52-year-old woman presented with shortness of breath, NYHA class II. She denies orthopnea and PND.

Her Cardiac Risk Factor was dyslipidemia. She had stage 3 of invasive ductal carcinoma of the left breast with lymph node metastatic disease, surgically treated with double mastectomy. She received adjuvant chemotherapy with doxorubicin, cyclophosphamide, four cycles, and paclitaxel plus trastuzumab three cycles. On examination she looks generally well, blood pressure 100/60 mmHg, and bi-basilar fine crackles on chest auscultation, heart has normal S1, S2 with a faint systolic murmur best heard in left lower sternal border, both lower extremities are symmetric in size, with no edema. A 12-lead electrocardiogram shows normal sinus rhythm with normal axis, heart rate of 69 bpm. She had normal myocardial perfusion scan.

Cycle four of paclitaxel plus trastuzumab was canceled because of an ejection fraction of 40% reported on echocardiogram. She was started on carvedilol and ramipril for heart failure with mid-range LVEF. Follow up echocardiogram showed LVEF improved to 53%, again she was started on Herceptin for 2 months, subsequently LVEF dropped again to 45% and Herceptin stopped permanently.

© The Author(s), under exclusive license to Springer Nature Switzerland AG 2021
A. Rohani, *Clinical Cases in Cardio-Oncology*, Clinical Cases in Cardiology, https://doi.org/10.1007/978-3-030-71155-9_7

Then she was started on tamoxifen, this also was discontinued. Patient started on triptorelin, Androgen-deprivation therapy (ADT) and she also completed radiotherapy.

On further follow up, patient has no symptoms suspicious for recurrence of her breast cancer, asymptomatic from cardiovascular standpoint and euvolemic on examination. Her LVEF also improved to 50% while on both carvedilol and ramipril.

Clinical Pearls

1. Trastuzumab-related cardiotoxicity is not related to cumulative dose. It is often reversible with treatment discontinuation, and re-challenge is often tolerated well after recovery.
2. Risk for heart failure may be limited by avoidance of concurrent use of doxorubicin dose exceeding 300 mg/m^2.
3. Risk factors of developing trastuzumab-related cardiotoxicity include previous or concurrent anthracycline use and age greater than 50 years and obesity: Risk of cardiotoxicity can be calculated by this equation [1]:

$$\frac{7 + (0.04 \times \text{age}) - (0.1 \times \text{baseline LVEF})}{4.76} \times 100$$

4. If the patient developed symptomatic heart failure, trastuzumab should be discontinued [2].
5. In the adjuvant setting, a baseline echocardiogram should be done with a repeat at 3, 6, 9, and 12 months [3].
6. In the metastatic setting, LVEF should be checked at baseline and then only in the presence of symptoms.
7. If the LVEF drops 16 or more percentage points from baseline or 10–15 percentage points from baseline to below the lower limit of normal, trastuzumab should be withheld for 4 weeks; at that point, LVEF is reassessed, and if LVEF remains below the normal level, trastuzumab must be discontinued permanently [4].

8. Trastuzumab-related cardiotoxicity is often reversible and responds well to management of heart failure. Many patients tolerate re-challenge [5].
9. Asymptomatic LVEF decline observed in up to 19% of patients receiving trastuzumab, however incidence of symptomatic heart failure reported from 2% to 4% [6].

References

1. Romond EH, Jeong JH, Rastogi P, Swain SM, Geyer CE Jr, Ewer MS, Rathi V, et al. Seven-year follow-up assessment of cardiac function in NSABP B-31, a randomized trial comparing doxorubicin and cyclophosphamide followed by paclitaxel (ACP) with ACP plus trastuzumab as adjuvant therapy for patients with node-positive, human epidermal growth factor receptor 2-positive breast cancer. J Clin Oncol. 2012;30(31):3792.
2. Henry ML, Niu J, Zhang N, Giordano SH, Chavez-MacGregor M. Cardiotoxicity and cardiac monitoring among chemotherapy-treated breast cancer patients. JACC Cardiovasc Imaging. 2018;11(8):1084–93. https://doi.org/10.1016/j.jcmg.2018.06.005.
3. Advani PP, Ballman KV, Dockter TJ, Colon-Otero G, Perez EA. Long-term cardiac safety analysis of NCCTG N9831 (Alliance) adjuvant trastuzumab trial. J Clin Oncol. 2016;34(6):581–7. https://doi.org/10.1200/JCO.2015.61.8413.
4. Bria E, Cuppone F, Fornier M, et al. Cardiotoxicity and incidence of brain metastases after adjuvant trastuzumab for early breast cancer: the dark side of the moon? A meta-analysis of the randomized trials. Breast Cancer Res Treat. 2008;109(2):231–9. https://doi.org/10.1007/s10549-007-9663-z.
5. Russell SD, Blackwell KL, Lawrence J, et al. Independent adjudication of symptomatic heart failure with the use of doxorubicin and cyclophosphamide followed by trastuzumab adjuvant therapy: a combined review of cardiac data from the National Surgical Adjuvant breast and Bowel Project B-31 and the North Central Cancer Treatment Group N9831 clinical trials. J Clin Oncol. 2010;28(21):3416–21. https://doi.org/10.1200/JCO.2009.23.6950.
6. Yu AF, Yadav NU, Lung BY, et al. Trastuzumab interruption and treatment-induced cardiotoxicity in early HER2-positive breast cancer. Breast Cancer Res Treat. 2015;149:489–95.

Chapter 8
Rituximab, Doxorubicin or Cancer Induced Tachycardia

Clinical Case

Patient was a 60-year-old woman with Follicular lymphoma Stage III, treated with Fludarabine and Rituximab for bulky cervical adenopathy. She then started on Rituxan, cyclophosphamide, doxorubicin, vincristine and prednisolone (R-CHOP) for six cycles. Patient complained of multiple episodes of palpitation occurred especially first day after first cycle of chemotherapy; Follow up Holter revealed multiple brief episodes of symptomatic NSVT (Fig. 8.1).

Laboratory tests showed normal electrolytes. An electrocardiogram (ECG) showed no ischemic changes, with normal QT interval. Echocardiogram revealed normal left ventricular size, systolic function and wall thickness, with no regional

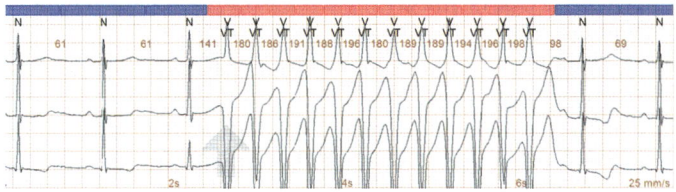

FIGURE 8.1 Non-sustained ventricular tachycardia on Holter

© The Author(s), under exclusive license to Springer Nature Switzerland AG 2021
A. Rohani, *Clinical Cases in Cardio-Oncology*, Clinical Cases in Cardiology, https://doi.org/10.1007/978-3-030-71155-9_8

wall motion abnormalities. Grade I/IV diastolic dysfunction (abnormal relaxation filling pattern), normal filling pressures. LVEF 63%. Global longitudinal strain: −20%, No significant valve abnormalities and normal left atrial volume index 32.4 ml/m². Myocardial perfusion scan revealed no evidence of ischemia.

She was started on metoprolol 25 mg twice daily. She again re-challenged with Rituxan for second cycle, this time under telemetry. No arrythmia occurred. She completed six cycles of R-CHOP and continued her treatment with Rituxan maintenance for 2 more years while she was on metoprolol. Follow up Holter monitor showed some brief episodes of asymptomatic supraventricular tachycardia but no episode of non-sustained ventricular tachycardia. After completion of Rituxan maintenance treatment, her lymphoma was in remission, metoprolol stopped and there was no recurrence of hemodynamically significant or symptomatic arrhythmia.

It is very hard to differentiate, if these episodes of NSVT were triggered by doxorubicin, Rituximab, cancer or a synergistic effect from all of these.

However, lack of LV dysfunction was against doxorubicin induced arrhythmia. Having said that, in the early phase of chemotherapy with doxorubicin, ECG changes and various arrythmias has been observed and reported.

Clinical Pearls [1–5]

- Arrhythmias have been reported in less than 1% of Rituximab infusions [1].
- Cardiac monitoring during and after the infusion in patients who develop clinically significant arrhythmias should be considered.
- There are case reports of arrythmia associated with rituximab infusion including AF and polymorphic ventricular tachycardia [1, 2].
- Rituximab administration is not associated with long-term cardiac toxicity.

- Patients with high circulating lymphocyte counts (>5000/µl) and structural heart disease are not recommended to receive more than 50 mg/h infusion of Rituxan [3].
- Any type of cancer can predispose patients to arrhythmia, because of inflammation and metabolic changes associated with cancer [4, 5].
- Obesity and alcohol use are risk factors for both cancer and arrythmia.

References

1. Poterucha JT, Westberg M, Nerheim P, Lovell JP. Rituximab-induced polymorphic ventricular tachycardia. Tex Heart Inst J. 2010;37(2):218–20.
2. Zamorano JL, Lancellotti P, Rodriguez Muñoz D, et al. 2016 ESC Position Paper on cancer treatments and cardiovascular toxicity developed under the auspices of the ESC Committee for Practice Guidelines: the Task Force for cancer treatments and cardiovascular toxicity of the European Society of Cardiology (ESC) [published correction appears in Eur Heart J. 2016 Dec 24]. Eur Heart J. 2016;37(36):2768–801.
3. Millward PM, Bandarenko N, Chang PP, et al. Cardiogenic shock complicates successful treatment of refractory thrombotic thrombocytopenia purpura with rituximab. Transfusion. 2005;45(9):1481–6. https://doi.org/10.1111/j.1537-2995.2005.00560.
4. Ostenfeld EB, Erichsen R, Pedersen L, Farkas DK, Weiss NS, Sørensen HT. Atrial fibrillation as a marker of occult cancer. PLoS One. 2014;9(8):e102861.
5. Buza V, Rajagopalan B, Curtis AB. Cancer treatment–induced arrhythmias. Circul Arrhyth Electrophysiol. 2017;10(8)

Chapter 9
Carfilzomib (CFZ) Induced Heart Failure with Reduced Ejection Fraction

Clinical Case

A 63-year-old female was diagnosed with Lambda light chain myeloma in the past 4 years, with acute kidney injury, requiring dialysis. Her cardiovascular risk factors include well controlled hypertension. She was treated with Cyclophosphamide + Bortezomib + Dexamethasone (CyBorD) for 12 cycles. Renal function improved with no ongoing requirement of dialysis. She again presented with left femur fracture 2 years later and bone marrow biopsy confirmed multiple myeloma relapse.

She was started on lenalidomide, dexamethasone and carfilzomib therapy. Two weeks later, she presented to the emergency department with shortness of breath, bilateral lung crackles and pitting edema on examination. Chest X ray showed pulmonary congestion. ECG has not changed in comparison with her baseline ECG. Troponin was negative two times with eight hours interval. Subsequent echocardiogram showed left ventricular ejection fraction of 32%. She was started on guideline-directed medical therapy (GDMT) of heart failure. CFZ treatment stopped and three months later, LVEF improved to 52%.

A. Rohani, *Clinical Cases in Cardio-Oncology*, Clinical Cases in Cardiology, https://doi.org/10.1007/978-3-030-71155-9_9

Clinical Pearls [1–5]

1. Carfilzomib (CFZ) induced heart failure with reduced ejection fraction has been reported in approximately 7% of patients particularly within the first 3 months of therapy. It is not dose dependent and there is no association with the duration of infusion [1, 2].
2. It is largely reversible, with prompt termination of treatment, however, rapidly progressing fatal heart failure is also reported [1].
3. Baseline ECG, Transthoracic echocardiogram should be considered in high risk patients.
4. Hypertension needs to be treated aggressively.
5. Education of patient and arrangement for tele home care including daily weight should be considered.
6. Repeat of echocardiogram in case of worsening symptoms should be considered [3, 4].
7. Coronary artery disease should be ruled out before making the diagnosis of Carfilzomib (CFZ) induced heart failure.
8. There must be low threshold for discontinuation of carfilzomib with any signs of cardiotoxicity [2–4].
9. Heart failure, and even death because of cardiac arrest has been reported even with 1 day of drug administration [2–4].
10. Known cardiovascular disease is risk factor for developing cardiotoxicity with Carfilzomib [5, 6].

References

1. Takakuwa T, Otomaru I, Araki T, et al. The first autopsy case of fatal acute cardiac failure after administration of carfilzomib in a patient with multiple myeloma. Case reports in hematology. 2019;(5)2019-24.
2. Siegel DS, Martin T, Wang M, et al. A phase 2 study of single-agent carfilzomib (PX-171-003-A1) in patients with relapsed and refractory multiple myeloma. Blood. 2012;120(14):2817–25. https://doi.org/10.1182/blood-2012-05-425934.

3. Grandin EW, Ky B, Cornell RF, Carver J, Lenihan DJ. Patterns of cardiac toxicity associated with irreversible proteasome inhibition in the treatment of multiple myeloma. J Card Fail. 2015;21(2):138–44.
4. Waxman AJ, Clasen S, Hwang WT, Garfall A, Vogl DT, Carver J, O'Quinn R, Cohen AD, Stadtmauer EA, Ky B, Weiss BM. Carfilzomib-associated cardiovascular adverse events: a systematic review and meta-analysis. JAMA Oncol. 2018;4(3):e174519. Epub 2018 Mar 8. PMID: 29285538; PMCID: PMC5885859. https://doi.org/10.1001/jamaoncol.2017.4519.
5. Dimopoulos MA, Roussou M, Gavriatopoulou M, Psimenou E, Ziogas D, Eleutherakis-Papaiakovou E, Fotiou D, Migkou M, Kanellias N, Panagiotidis I, Ntalianis A, Papadopoulou E, Stamatelopoulos K, Manios E, Pamboukas C, Kontogiannis S, Terpos E, Kastritis E. Cardiac and renal complications of carfilzomib in patients with multiple myeloma. Blood Adv. 2017;1(7):449–54. PMID: 29296960; PMCID: PMC5738981. https://doi.org/10.1182/bloodadvances.2016003269.
6. Cornell RF, Ky B, Weiss BM, Dahm CN, Gupta DK, Du L, Carver JR, Cohen AD, Engelhardt BG, Garfall AL, Goodman SA, Harrell SL, Kassim AA, Jadhav T, Jagasia M, Moslehi J, O'Quinn R, Savona MR, Slosky D, Smith A, Stadtmauer EA, Vogl DT, Waxman A, Lenihan D. Prospective study of cardiac events during proteasome inhibitor therapy for relapsed multiple myeloma. J Clin Oncol. 2019;37(22):1946–55. Epub 2019 Jun 12. PMID: 31188726. https://doi.org/10.1200/JCO.19.00231.

Chapter 10
Immune Checkpoint Inhibitor Cardiovascular Toxicities

Clinical Case

Patient was a 58 years old woman who was diagnosed 6 years ago with metastatic non-small cell lung adenocarcinoma, treated with surgical resection, concurrent radiation therapy of 30 Gray in 10 fractions, chemotherapy with cisplatin and etoposide; followed by maintenance pemetrexed.

Two years later, she was diagnosed with recurrence in the lungs and liver. She was started on first-line palliative immunotherapy with nivolumab, (anti-programmed cell death receptor 1) with excellent clinical response and tolerance.

She presented with one episode of unwitnessed syncope while she was sitting with no prodromes. Physical examination was unremarkable with no evidence of orthostatic hypotension.

ECG showed normal sinus rhythm and new bi-fascicular block. (right bundle branch block and left anterior fascicular block)

Patient was not anemic and had normal TSH but elevated troponin and BNP. Given new ECG changes, presence of syncope, and elevated troponin, patient diagnosed with immune checkpoint inhibitor myocarditis and Nivolumab stopped. A coronary angiogram was done, and coronary arteries were normal.

© The Author(s), under exclusive license to Springer Nature Switzerland AG 2021
A. Rohani, *Clinical Cases in Cardio-Oncology*, Clinical Cases in Cardiology, https://doi.org/10.1007/978-3-030-71155-9_10

Echocardiogram revealed normal left ventricular size and wall thickness. Left ventricular ejection fraction was mildly impaired and estimated at 50%. Right ventricular size and function appeared normal. There was mild aortic valve regurgitation and mild mitral valve regurgitation. Cardiovascular magnetic resonance (CMR) confirmed diagnosis of myocarditis.

Patient was started on high dose intravenous methylprednisolone (1000 mg/day for 3 days), with progressive tapering. The patient's troponin levels trended down quickly.

The ejection fraction improved and on follow up patient is doing well from cardiovascular standpoint, however was not started back on Nivolumab.

Clinical Pearls

1. Prevalence of immune checkpoint inhibitor myocarditis is between 0.06% and 2.4%. The onset is within 3 months of treatment initiation in 81% of cases. It could occur even after 1–2 doses of immunotherapy [1].
2. Presentations of cardiotoxicity include: Acute coronary syndrome, atherosclerosis progression, new-onset heart failure even cardiogenic shock, and chronic heart failure. Pericardial disease, recurrent pericardial and pleural effusions, Takotsubo cardiomyopathy, venous thromboembolism, conduction abnormalities, arrhythmias, syncope, and even sudden cardiac death has also been reported.
3. Risk factors:

    (a) Combination of ICI therapy with other cardiotoxic treatment like as use of anthracyclines.
    (b) Underlying cardiovascular disease or autoimmune disease could be a risk factor, however a depressed LVEF is not a requirement for cardiotoxicity.
    (c) ICI-related skeletal myositis
    (d) Genetic factors.

4. In patients treated with the combination of nivolumab plus ipilimumab incidence of myocarditis is higher compared with nivolumab alone (0.27 vs. 0.06%).

Diagnosis of ICI-Associated Myocarditis [1–4]

Role of screening for myocarditis is unknown, however, baseline ECG and measurement of serum troponin are recommended. If ICI-induced cardiotoxicity is suspected, ICI therapy should be withheld. Figure 10.1 summarizes an anecdotal evidence and expert opinion recommendation approach for patients receiving immune checkpoint inhibitors [1–4].

- In asymptomatic cases, if myocarditis is confirmed, serum erythrocyte sedimentation rate, C-reactive protein, C3, and C4 should be measured.
- Troponin: Almost always is increased in the setting of myocarditis.

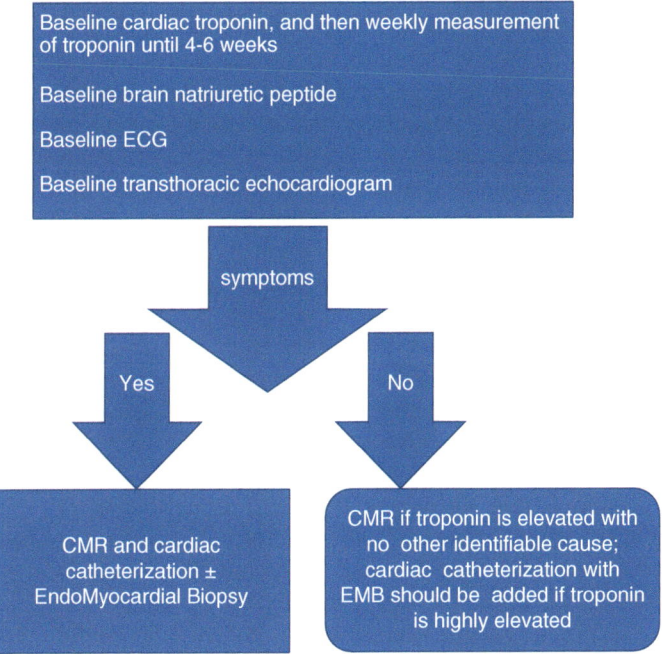

FIGURE 10.1 Anecdotal evidence and expert opinion recommendation approach for patients receiving immune checkpoint inhibitors [1–4]. *CMR* cardiovascular magnetic resonance imaging, *EMB* endo myocardial biopsy

- Electrocardiogram (ECG): findings are non-specific. New ECG changes/new arrythmia should be considered abnormal.
- Echocardiography is useful for determining cardiac function but not for definite diagnosis of myocarditis. Echo findings in favor of myocarditis include presence of wall motion abnormalities or LVEF < 50%.
- In a recent study published in Journal of American College of Cardiology by Awadalla M et al., it was showed that GLS declines in ICI myocarditis. It also revealed that, during follow-up, patients with low GLS are at higher risk to develop major adverse cardiac events (MACE) [5].
- Definitive imaging modality is cardiac magnetic resonance (CMR).
- Endomyocardial biopsy (EMB)is the gold standard of diagnosis with risk of major complication at <1% in experienced centers. To reduce false-negative result, at least six samples should be gathered. It was suggested, as the CMR has acceptable sensitivity and specificity for diagnosis of myocarditis, there is no need to perform endomyocardial biopsy routinely, especially in unstable patients or in the context of severe thrombocytopenia. Histological finding is mostly a T-cell–predominant lymphocytic infiltrate which is like acute allograft rejection in cardiac transplant patients.
- Diagnosis of ICI myocarditis is mostly a diagnosis of exclusion based on the level of suspicion for myocarditis.

Grading [6–10]:
- G1: subclinical myocarditis (abnormal troponin/creatine kinase/Brain Natriuretic Peptide or abnormal ECG).
- G2: Mild symptoms and abnormal troponin/creatine kinase/Brain Natriuretic Peptide and abnormal ECG
- G3: Symptomatic and clinically stable cases (abnormal troponin/creatine kinase/Brain Natriuretic Peptide and abnormal ECG, LVEF < 50% or wall motion abnormality on echocardiogram, cardiac MRI diagnostic or suggestive)

- G4: Decompensated unstable patients, life threatening disease with abnormal echocardiogram, abnormal CMR, elevated troponin/creatine kinase/Brain Natriuretic Peptide and abnormal ECG.

Management of ICI-Associated Myocarditis
- Holding checkpoint inhibitor therapy is recommended for all grades of complications (including asymptomatic isolated rise in troponin) [11].
- At this time, there is no consistent approach for management; all-grade toxicities should have early administration of high-dose corticosteroids (1 mg/kg daily of either intravenous or oral steroids) and tapering over at least 4–6 weeks). In a recent study, published in Circulation, it was suggested that rapid start and higher initial dose of corticosteroid (i.e., intravenous methylprednisolone 1000 mg/day) is associated with rapid regaining of left ventricular function and reducing the number of MACE [11, 12].
- If there is no immediate response to high-dose corticosteroids, rejection doses of corticosteroids (methylprednisolone 1 g every day) and the addition of infliximab, antithymocyte globulin, mycophenolate, or abatacept should be considered. There is a case report published in New England Journal of Medicine, which showed successful treatment of severe, glucocorticoid-refractory myocarditis induced by an immune checkpoint inhibitor, with abatacept (approved for use in patients with rheumatic diseases). It was concluded that abatacept could lead to inactivation of the normal immune response [13, 14].
- In the Presence of symptoms and if there is hemodynamic instability patient needs to be admitted in CCU and transferred to a heart transplant facility.

Re-challenge:
- There is one case report in a patient with nivolumab myocarditis re-challenged with a different ICI, pembrolizumab, who developed worsening heart failure 2 weeks after the first dose [9].

- American Society of Clinical Oncology Guidelines recommend permanently discontinuing ICI for Grade 2 toxicity or higher [12, 13, 15].

References

1. Ganatra S, Neilan TG. Immune checkpoint inhibitor associated myocarditis. Oncologist. 2018;23:518–23.
2. Mahmood SS, Fradley MG, Cohen JV, Nohria A, Reynolds KL, Heinzerling LM, et al. Myocarditis in patients treated with immune checkpoint inhibitors. J Am Coll Cardiol. 2018;71(16):1755–64.
3. Moslehi JJ, Salem JE, Sosman JA, Lebrun-Vignes B, Johnson DB. Increased reporting of fatal immune checkpoint inhibitor-associated myocarditis. Lancet. 2018;391(10124):933.
4. Johnson DB, Balko JM, Compton ML, et al. Fulminant myocarditis with combination immune checkpoint blockade. N Engl J Med. 2016;375:1749–55.
5. Awadalla M, Mahmood SS, Groarke JD, Hassan MZO, Nohria A, Rokicki A, et al. Global longitudinal strain and cardiac events in patients with immune checkpoint inhibitor-related myocarditis. J Am Coll Cardiol. 2020;75:467–78.
6. Palaskas N, Lopez-Mattei J, Durand JB, Iliescu C, Deswal A. Immune Checkpoint inhibitor myocarditis: pathophysiological characteristics, diagnosis, and treatment. J Am Heart Assoc. 2020;9(2):e013757. doi:https://doi.org/10.1161/JAHA.119.013757. Heinzerling et al., Journal for Immunotherapy of Cancer, 2017;29, 136–144.
7. Varricchi G, Galdiero MR, Marone G, Criscuolo G, Triassi M, Bonaduce D, Marone G, Tocchetti CG. Cardiotoxicity of immune checkpoint inhibitors. ESMO Open. 2017;26;2(4):e000247.
8. Moslehi JJ. Immune checkpoint inhibitor-associated cardiotoxicities: Learning from mice and humans [abstract]. In: Proceedings of the AACR Special Conference on Tumor Immunology and Immunotherapy, Boston, MA, 2019 Nov 17–20. Philadelphia, PA: AACR; Cancer Immunol Res 2020;8(3 Suppl):Abstract nr IA10.
9. Tajmir-Riahi A, Bergmann T, Schmid M, Agaimy A, Schuler G, Heinzerling L. Life-threatening autoimmune cardiomyopathy reproducibly induced in a patient by checkpoint inhibitor therapy. J Immunother. 2018;41:35–8.

10. Behling J, Kaes J, Munzel T, Grabbe S, Loquai C. New-onset third-degree atrioventricular block because of autoimmune-induced myositis under treatment with anti-programmed cell death-1 (nivolumab) for metastatic melanoma. Melanoma Res. 2017;27:155–8.

11. Brahmer JR, Lacchetti C, Schneider BJ, et al. Management of immune-related adverse events in patients treated with immune checkpoint inhibitor therapy: American Society of Clinical Oncology Clinical Practice Guideline. J Clin Oncol. 2018;36:1714–68.

12. Zhang L, Zlotoff DA, Awadalla M, Mahmood SS, Nohria A, Hassan MZO, et al. Major adverse cardiovascular events and the timing and dose of corticosteroids in immune checkpoint inhibitor-associated Myocarditis. Circulation. 2020;141(24):2031–4. Epub 2020 Jun 15. PMID: 32539614; PMCID: PMC7301778. https://doi.org/10.1161/CIRCULATIONAHA.119.044703.

13. Geraud A, Gougis P, Vozy A, et al. Clinical pharmacology and interplay of immune checkpoint agents: a Yin-Yang balance. Annu Rev Pharmacol Toxicol. 2020; [Epub ahead of print].

14. Salem JE, Allenbach Y, Vozy A, Brechot N, Johnson DB, Moslehi JJ, Kerneis M. Abatacept for severe immune checkpoint inhibitor-associated myocarditis. N Engl J Med. 2019;380(24):2377–9.

15. https://www.acc.org/latest-in-cardiology/articles/2020/10/30/15/06/diagnosis-and-treatment-of-immune-checkpoint-inhibitor-associated-myocarditis-and-acs?utm_medium=social&utm_source=twitter_post&utm_campaign=twitter_post

Chapter 11
Androgen Deprivation Therapy Cardiotoxicity

Clinical Case

The patient is a 63-year-old male, case of metastatic castrate-sensitive prostate cancer on goserelin injections every 3 month. His past medical history was significant for hypertension and hyperlipidemia. He denies any cardiovascular-related symptoms.

On examination, he looks generally well, alert and oriented ×3. Blood pressure 130/85 mmHg, pulse rate of 74 bpm and oxygen saturation of 96% on room air. Chest is clear, there are no adventitious sounds, heart has normal S1, S2, with no murmur. Given his initial Gleason [1] grade of 8, as well as doubling PSA in 7 months since starting treatment, he was started on androgen receptor inhibitor, apalutamide. Two weeks after starting treatment with apalutamide, patient presented with chest pain and shortness of breath.

He had an echocardiogram, which showed an ejection fraction of LVEF: 46%. Coronary angiogram showed moderate diffuse coronary artery disease but no significant obstruction.

He was provided with betablocker, aspirin, and ramipril.

This event could be explained by his underlying risk factors, triggered by apalutamide and ADT. He has had an excellent response to apalutamide treatment, and his most recent

A. Rohani, *Clinical Cases in Cardio-Oncology*, Clinical Cases in Cardiology, https://doi.org/10.1007/978-3-030-71155-9_11

PSA was down to 0.15 mcg/L. He has been medically optimized for HFmrEF and follow up echocardiogram showed improvement in his LV systolic function.

Clinical Pearls

Risk of treatment with ADT:

1. There is an increased risk of diabetes and cardiovascular disease with ADT but there is no significant increase in risk of cardiovascular death. Apalutamide could increase risk of hypertension [2–5].

2. Higher risk of thromboembolic diseases (pulmonary, arterial embolism and deep venous thrombosis) also described with ADT [6, 7].

3. ADT can prolong the QT/QTc interval (modest risk for apalutamide) [8].

Higher risk for cardiovascular events observed in patients with:

• Two or more prior cardiovascular disease events.
• First six months after initiation of ADT

Aggressive management of hyperlipidemia, hypertension, diabetes mellitus [9], and smoking cessation as well as three or more hours of aerobic physical activity per week is strongly recommended [7].

The risk for cardiovascular disease may be lower in patients treated with GnRH antagonists in compare to other forms of ADT. Table 11.1 summarizes different ADT drugs with their mechanism of action, Table 11.2 summarizes major side effects with different types of ADT [10, 11].

TABLE 11.1 Different ADT drugs with their mechanism of action

GnRH agonists	Leuprolide
	Goserelin
GnRH antagonists	Degarelix
17-α-hydroxylase inhibitor	Abiraterone
Androgen receptor inhibitor	Apalutamide

TABLE 11.2 Major side effects with different types of ADT

Abiraterone	1. Fluid retention
	2. Hypertension
	3. Cardiac arrhythmia
	4. Patients need to be closely monitored at least monthly for hypertension, hypokalemia, and fluid retention.
	5. May increase the serum concentration of Carvedilol and Metoprolol.
Leuprolide	QT-prolongation
Apalutamide	1. Myocardial infarction
	2. May decrease the serum concentration of Ticagrelor, Rivaroxaban, Digoxin, Dabigatran
	3. May increase serum concentrations of Clopidogrel
	4. Discontinuing apalutamide therapy should be considered for grade 3 or 4 of ischemic cardiovascular events.
	5. Concentration-dependent increase in QTc is also observed

References

1. Bostwick DG. Gleason grading of prostatic needle biopsies. Correlation with grade in 316 matched prostatectomies. Am J Surg Pathol. 1994;18(8):796–803.
2. Iacovelli R, Ciccarese C, Bria E, et al. The cardiovascular toxicity of abiraterone and enzalutamide in prostate cancer. Clin Genitourin Cancer. 2018;16(3):e645–53.
3. Higano CS. Cardiovascular disease and androgen axis-targeted drugs for prostate cancer. N Engl J Med. 2020;382(23):2257–9.

4. Nguyen PL, Je Y, Schutz FA, et al. Association of androgen deprivation therapy with cardiovascular death in patients with prostate cancer: a meta-analysis of randomized trials. JAMA. 2011;306(21):2359–66.

5. Schmitt CA. Urological cancer: heart facts rehabilitate ADT. Nat Rev Clin Oncol. 2012;9(2):68.

6. Van Hemelrijck M, Adolfsson J, Garmo H, et al. Risk of thromboembolic diseases in men with prostate cancer: results from the population-based PCBaSe Sweden. Lancet Oncol. 2010;11(5):450–8.

7. Ehdaie B, Atoria CL, Gupta A, et al. Androgen deprivation and thromboembolic events in men with prostate cancer. Cancer. 2012;118(13):3397–406.

8. Gardner JR, Livingston PM, Fraser SF. Effects of exercise on treatment-related adverse effects for patients with prostate cancer receiving androgen-deprivation therapy: a systematic review. J Clin Oncol. 2014;32(4):335–46.

9. Keating NL, O'Malley AJ, Freedland SJ, Smith MR. Diabetes and cardiovascular disease during androgen deprivation therapy: observational study of veterans with prostate cancer [published correction appears in J Natl Cancer Inst. 2012 Oct 3;104(19):1518-23]. J Natl Cancer Inst. 2010;102(1):39–46. https://doi.org/10.1093/jnci/djp404.

10. Saigal CS, Gore JL, Krupski TL, et al. Androgen deprivation therapy increases cardiovascular morbidity in men with prostate cancer. Cancer. 2007;110(7):1493–500. https://doi.org/10.1002/cncr.22933.

11. Smith MR, Saad F, Chowdhury S, Oudard S, Hadaschik B, Graff JN, Olmos D, Mainwaring PN, Lee JY, Uemura H, et al. Apalutamide treatment and metastasis-free survival in prostate cancer. N Engl J Med. 2018;378:1408–18.

Chapter 12
5-FU Induced Atrial Fibrillation in the Context of Ischemic Heart Disease

Clinical Case

Patient was a 71-year-old male with metastatic HER2-negative gastric adenocarcinoma, and placement of gastric stent, previously on FOLFOX chemotherapy with oxaliplatin cessation due to painful neuropathy, currently on modified de Gramont 5-FU. His past medical history was significant of liver transplant, Hepatitis C and diabetes. He presented three times to the Emergency department with a rapid heart rate. He was found to be in atrial fibrillation (Fig. 12.1) with heart rate of 160 beats per minute. One time, he received verapamil 2.5 mg IV. With this, he converted to normal sinus rhythm. He was started on direct oral anticoagulation and Verapamil, Extended release, 180 mg once daily; He again presented to the hospital following another chemotherapy with 5-FU. On this presentation to the emergency department, he had troponin rise associated with chest tightness. On examination, he had blood pressure of 142/49 mmHg, pulse rate of 120 beats per minute, irregularly irregular, respiratory rate 16 per minute, oxygen saturation of 99% on room air. JVP was flat. Chest was clear. No adventitious sound. Heart had normal S1, S2, irregularly irregular with no murmur. Both lower extremities were symmetric in size with no edema. He underwent successful electrical cardioversion.

© The Author(s), under exclusive license to Springer Nature Switzerland AG 2021
A. Rohani, *Clinical Cases in Cardio-Oncology*, Clinical Cases in Cardiology, https://doi.org/10.1007/978-3-030-71155-9_12

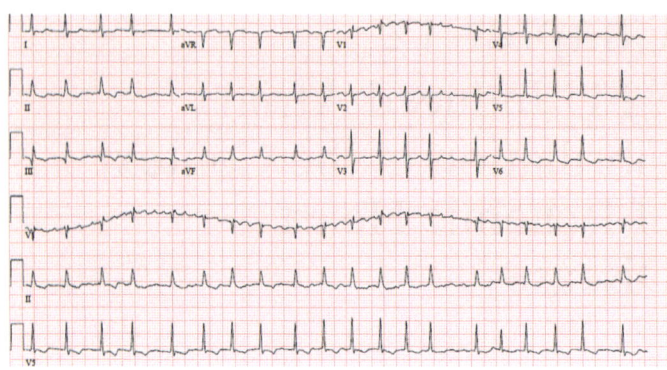

FIGURE 12.1 Atrial fibrillation with HR:120 bpm

While admitted in hospital, given raise in troponin and to rule out ischemia as the underlying mechanism of recurrent AF as well as chemotherapy with 5-FU, he underwent coronary angiogram which showed: Diffuse coronary artery disease.

80% stenosis in the mid LAD. 80% stenosis in the proximal RCA with diffuse distal disease.

He underwent successful PCI of the mid LAD and proximal RCA. After PCI, there was no recurrence of clinical AF.

We think the occurrence of AF in this patient was multifactorial due to a combination of his underlying comorbidities, coronary artery disease triggered by 5FU.

Clinical Pearls

- CAD and AF are ugly sisters [2]: CAD commonly seen in AF patients with 17–46% prevalence.
- The occurrence of AF in cancer patients are multifactorial: a combination of inflammation, direct action of cancer and the adverse side effects of anticancer agents.
- Atrial branch (originate from the Right Coronary Artery) occlusion and Atrial ischemia is an independent predictor of new-onset AF observed in many studies. 5-FU induced

arterial vasocontraction aggravates ischemia and is a leading cause of AF [3].

- Coronary-dilating agents along with PCI should be considered for treatment of AF which occurs after the administration of 5-FU and is refractory to antiarrhythmic agents [4].
- Food and Drug Administration (FDA) approved uridine triacetate as an antidote to 5-FU or capecitabine. Indications include [5, 6]
  - Early-onset, life-threatening cardiac or central nervous system toxicity.
  - Severe gastrointestinal toxicity and/or neutropenia.
- Daily administration of capecitabine and continuous infusion of 5FU, has the same risk of cardiotoxicity around 3–9% (higher incidence reported in patients treated with combine treatment of capecitabine, oxaliplatin and bevacizumab around 12%) [7].
- Cardiotoxicity presentations include: Acute coronary syndrome, diffuse pleuritic pain, transient asymptomatic bradycardia, Arrhythmias like as AF, Acute pulmonary edema, Cardiac arrest and Pericarditis [8].
- Bolus injection of 5-FU has fewer side effects in comparison to infusional regimen (incidence of cardiotoxicity is between 1.6 and 3% in contrast to 2–18% risk with continuous infusional regimens of 5 days or longer) [9].
- Suggested Risk factors for fluoropyrimidine cardiotoxicity include older age, concomitant radiotherapy, other cardiotoxic chemotherapy exposure, and underlying heart disease, however there is conflicting available data insufficient for justify or withholding treatment [10].
- Timeline: Cardiotoxicity most commonly happens during the first cycle of treatment mostly in first 12 hours following infusion (with a range between 3 and 18 hours) [11].
- For most patients with suspected fluoropyrimidine-induced chest pain, diagnostic coronary arteriography is indicated to exclude another concomitant process that could account for an acute coronary syndrome.
- Fluoropyrimidine-induced cardiotoxicity is not dose dependent.

- QTc interval should be monitored. High risk: >10% incidence of long QT with capecitabine treatment reported [12].

Re-challenge:
- If it is not feasible to switch to a non-fluoropyrimidine chemotherapy or benefit of 5-FU in treatment of cancer is estimated to be more than the risk of cardiotoxicity, re-challenge could be considered with following precautionary measurement:
- Detailed informed consent should be obtained from patients. Careful observation on an inpatient unit with continuous ECG monitoring are advisable during drug infusion [13].
- Pretreatment for at least 48 hours with aspirin and both a calcium channel blocker (diltiazem starting at 90 mg twice daily and titrated to 180 mg twice daily, if tolerated) and nitrates (isosorbide dinitrate up titrated to the highest possible dose based upon blood pressure) are recommended.
- 5-FU administration should be immediately discontinued if any symptoms or signs of acute cardiac event occurred [14, 15].
- Beta-blockers should be avoided, given concerns for unopposed alpha receptor activation in any situation of potential increased adrenergic state (e.g., pain, anxiety) [16, 17].

References

1. de Gramont A, Krulik M, Cady J, Lagadec B, Maisani JE, Loiseau JP, Grange JD, Gonzalez-Canali G, Demuynck B, Louvet C. High-dose leucovorin and 5-fluorouracil bolus and infusion in advanced colorectal cancer. Eur J Clin Oncol. 1988;24:1499–503.
2. Michniewicz E, Mlodawska E, Lopatowska P, Tomaszuk-Kazberuk A, Malyszko J. Patients with atrial fibrillation and coronary artery disease — double trouble. Adv Med Sci. 2018;63:30–5.
3. Alasady M, Abhayaratna W, Leong DP, Lim HS, Abed HS, Brooks AG, et al. Coronary artery disease affecting the atrial

branches is an independent determinant of atrial fibrillation after myocardial infarction. Heart Rhythm. 2011;8:955–60.

4. Insights into onco-cardiology: atrial fibrillation in cancer. J Am Coll Cardiol. 2014;63:945–53. https://www.sciencedirect.com/science/article/pii/S0735109713063559

5. Kondo Y, Kobayashi Y. New-onset atrial fibrillation after atrial ischemia. J Arrhythm. 2019;35(6):863–4. https://doi.org/10.1002/joa3.12233.

6. Moriyama S, Yokoyama T, Irie K, et al. Atrial fibrillation observed in a patient with esophageal cancer treated with fluorouracil. J Cardiol Cases. 2019;20(5):183–6. https://doi.org/10.1016/j.jccase.2019.08.005.

7. Zamorano JL, Lancellotti P, Rodriguez Muñoz D, Aboyans V, Asteggiano R, Galderisi M. 2016 ESC Position Paper on cancer treatments and cardiovascular toxicity developed under the auspices of the ESC Committee for Practice Guidelines. Eur Heart J. 2016;37:2768–801.

8. Labianca R, Beretta G, Clerici M, Fraschini P, Luporini G. Cardiac toxicity of 5-fluorouracil: a study on 1083 patients. Tumori. 1982;68(6):505–10.

9. Anand AJ. Fluorouracil cardiotoxicity. Ann Pharmacother. 1994;28(3):374–8.

10. Gaveau T, Banzet P, Marneffe H, Viars P. Trobules cardio-vasculaires au cours d'infections d'anti-mitotiques à fortes doses. 30 observations cliniques [Cardiovascular disorders in the course of antimitotic infusions at high doses. 30 clinical cases]. Anesth Analg (Paris). 1969;26(3):311–27.

11. Saif MW, Shah MM, Shah AR. Fluoropyrimidine-associated cardiotoxicity: revisited. Expert Opin Drug Saf. 2009;8(2):191–202. https://doi.org/10.1517/14740330902733961.

12. Jensen SA, Hasbak P, Mortensen J, Sørensen JB. Fluorouracil induces myocardial ischemia with increases of plasma brain natriuretic peptide and lactic acid but without dysfunction of left ventricle. J Clin Oncol. 2010;28(36):5280–6. https://doi.org/10.1200/JCO.2009.27.3953.

13. Tsibiribi P, Descotes J, Lombard-Bohas C, et al. Cardiotoxicity of 5-fluorouracil in 1350 patients with no prior history of heart disease. Bull Cancer. 2006;93(3):E27–30.

14. Lestuzzi C, Vaccher E, Talamini R, et al. Effort myocardial ischemia during chemotherapy with 5-fluorouracil: an underestimated risk. Ann Oncol. 2014;25(5):1059–64. https://doi.org/10.1093/annonc/mdu055.

15. Kwakman JJ, Simkens LH, Mol L, Kok WE, Koopman M, Punt CJ. Incidence of capecitabine-related cardiotoxicity in different treatment schedules of metastatic colorectal cancer: a retrospective analysis of the CAIRO studies of the Dutch Colorectal Cancer Group. Eur J Cancer. 2017;76:93–9.
16. Polk A, Vaage-Nilsen M, Vistisen K, Nielsen DL. Cardiotoxicity in cancer patients treated with 5-fluorouracil or capecitabine: a systematic review of incidence, manifestations and predisposing factors. Cancer Treat Rev. 2013;39(8):974–84.
17. de Forni M, Malet-Martino MC, Jaillais P, et al. Cardiotoxicity of high-dose continuous infusion fluorouracil: a prospective clinical study. J Clin Oncol. 1992;10(11):1795–801. https://doi.org/10.1200/JCO.1992.10.11.1795.

Chapter 13
Cisplatin Induced Acute Coronary Syndrome

Clinical Case

Patient was a 35-year-old male presented with painless swelling of right testicle. Scrotal ultrasound revealed well-defined hypoechoic lesions without cystic areas. He was diagnosed with stage IIB Testicular germ-cell cancer (TGCC). He was non-smoker and had no other cardiovascular risk factors. His body mass index was 28 kg/m². He was started on four cycle of Bleomycin, Etoposide and Cisplatin (BEP) therapy. Ten days after cycle four, he presented with severe crescendo retrosternal chest pain at rest to the emergency department. On examination, patient had blood pressure of 163/100 mmHg, heart rate of 123 bpm, cardiac exam revealed normal S1, S2 and S3 gallop, on chest auscultation he had bilateral basal fine crackles, both lower extremities were symmetric in size with no edema. Electrocardiogram showed significant ST segment depression in anterior leads. (Wellens syndrome, Fig. 13.1, deep T wave inversion in anterior leads which is specific for proximal stenosis of the left anterior descending (LAD) coronary artery [1]. Coronary angiogram revealed proximal of the left anterior descending (LAD) artery had 95% stenosis. Patient underwent thrombus aspiration and percutaneous coronary intervention performed with a drug eluting stent.

© The Author(s), under exclusive license to Springer Nature Switzerland AG 2021
A. Rohani, *Clinical Cases in Cardio-Oncology*, Clinical Cases in Cardiology, https://doi.org/10.1007/978-3-030-71155-9_13

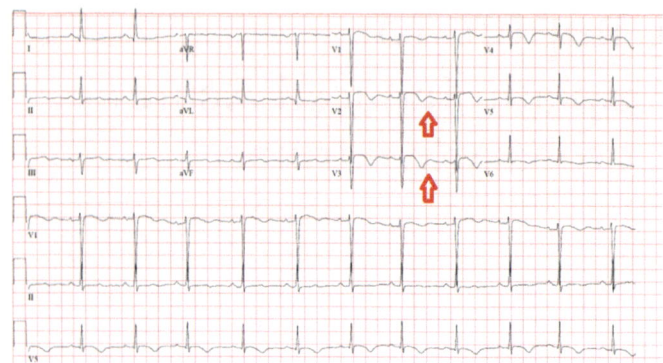

FIGURE 13.1   Red arrows shows deep T inversion, Wellens syndrome

Clinical Pearls

Higher Risk of vascular events with cisplatin [2]:

1. Higher-accumulated dose of cisplatin therapy and radiation therapy (RT).
2. Body mass index >25 kg/m², presence of other cardiovascular risk factors like as: smoking, HTN, hyperlipidemia, and DM.

   Increase in incidence of Deep vein thrombosis and pulmonary embolism [3]:

1. Body surface area >1.9 m²
2. Elevated lactate dehydrogenase (LDH).

   Mechanism of vascular events with cisplatin: impairment of endothelium dependent vasodilatation and acute coronary thrombosis.

   Other Side effects with cisplatin [4, 5]:

   Metabolic syndrome—close monitoring of lipid profile (mostly increase in low-density lipoprotein) and blood pressure recommended. Patients receiving more than 850 mg of cisplatin are especially at risk of developing HTN. Insulin resistance and obesity also reported as side effects of Cisplatin chemotherapy.

References

1. de Zwaan C, Bär FW, Wellens HJ. Characteristic electrocardio-graphic pattern indicating a critical stenosis high in left anterior descending coronary artery in patients admitted because of impending myocardial infarction. Am Heart J. 1982;103(4 Pt 2):730–6.
2. van den Belt-Dusebout AW, Nuver J, de Wit R, et al. Long-term risk of cardiovascular disease in 5-year survivors of testicular cancer. J Clin Oncol. 2006;24(3):467–75.
3. Fung C, Fossa SD, Milano MT, Sahasrabudhe DM, Peterson DR, Travis LB. Cardiovascular disease mortality after chemotherapy or surgery for testicular nonseminoma: a population-based study. J Clin Oncol. 2015;33(28):3105–15.
4. Lauritsen J, Hansen MK, Bandak M, et al. Cardiovascular risk factors and disease after male germ cell cancer. J Clin Oncol. 2020;38(6):584–92.
5. Herrmann J. Vascular toxic effects of cancer therapies. Nat Rev Cardiol. 2020;17:503–22.

Chapter 14
Radiotherapy and Valvular Heart Disease

Clinical Case

Patient was a 76-year-old female presented with worsening shortness of breath, both at rest and with exertion. She denies orthopnea, chest pain and syncope.

Her Cardiac Risk Factors include Diabetes, Hyperlipidemia and Hypertension.

Her Past Medical History was significant for bilateral breast cancer with involvement of the right supraclavicular lymph node, treated with bilateral mastectomies followed by chest wall and regional lymph node radiation ×50 fractions, completed 12 years ago. There was no history of chemotherapy for breast cancer. There has not been evidence of breast cancer recurrence.

On examination she looks generally well, blood pressure 130/80 mmHg, chest was clear. There was no adventitious sound, heart had normal S1, S2 with grade 3/6 systolic murmur, more prominent in aortic valve area, and diastolic murmur in apical area, both lower extremities were symmetric in size with no edema.

Echocardiogram showed aorto-mitral curtain thickening and calcification, moderate Aortic valve Stenosis (mean pressure gradient of 25 mmHg, LVOT to aortic valve velocity ratio of 0.32) severe mitral annular calcification and mitral

A. Rohani, *Clinical Cases in Cardio-Oncology*, Clinical Cases in Cardiology, https://doi.org/10.1007/978-3-030-71155-9_14

valve Stenosis, mean pressure gradient 13 mmHg at the heart rate of 82 bpm, mild to moderate MR, normal LV size and systolic function and mitral valve area of 0.8 cm^2.

A 12-lead electrocardiogram showed normal sinus rhythm with normal axis and heart rate of 82 bpm, voltage criteria for LVH and occasional premature atrial contraction (PAC).

She had Normal coronary angiogram. With this background, she was referred to Cardiac Surgery/Heart Valve Team for further assessment and possible treatment.

She was turned down for cardiac surgery as calcification was remarkably extensive, and operation considered to be prohibitively hazardous given the fact that she will require extensive mitral valve decalcification and reconstruction of the posterior annulus. One year later, she was diagnosed with moderately differentiated hepatocellular carcinoma, underwent Radiofrequency ablation of liver lesion and currently she is on observation.

Clinical Pearls

1. Pericarditis is the typical acute manifestation of radiation injury, however with newer radiation protocols, it is less common but there is risk of constrictive pericarditis due to inflammation and fibrosis, several years after radiation. The strongest risk factor for toxicity is the mean dose of radiation to the pericardium [1, 2].
2. Coronary artery disease: It is typically diffuse and extensively calcified. Screening with stress test or cardiac CT scan is suggested for high risk patients [3, 4].
3. Cardiomyopathy: chemotherapy with anthracycline increases risk of cardiomyopathy [5].
4. Valvular disease: fibrotic changes and calcification has been observed, mostly on the left side valves. In one study, aorto-mitral curtain thickening (Fig. 14.1) was reported as a marker of previous heart irradiation and mortality in patients undergoing cardiovascular surgery [6].
5. Conduction abnormalities: Fibrosis of conduction system, years or decades after the original treatment could lead to subsequent arrhythmias [7].

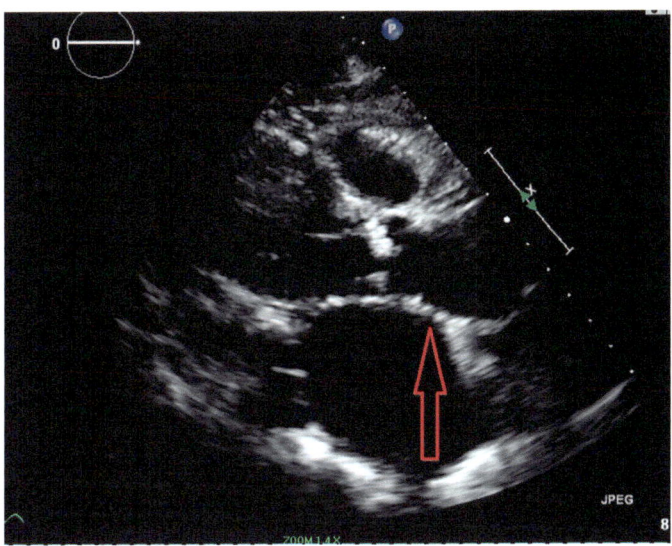

FIGURE 14.1 Red arrow shows aorto-mitral curtain thickening and calcification: a marker of previous heart irradiation

6. There is no safe minimum radiation dose.
7. Time: Cardiovascular events happen mostly within the first 5 years after treatment, but risk can remain elevated for 20 years after [8].
8. Risk: Patients with cardiovascular risk factors (hypertension, hyperlipidemia, smoking) and previous history of cardiovascular disease are at increased risk of cardiotoxicity following RT [9].

References

1. Moslehi J. The cardiovascular perils of cancer survivorship. N Engl J Med. 2013;368(11):1055–6. PMID: 23484833. https://doi.org/10.1056/NEJMe1215300.
2. Travis LB, Ng AK, Allan JM, Pui CH, Kennedy AR, Xu XG, Purdy JA, Applegate K, Yahalom J, Constine LS, Gilbert ES, Boice JD Jr. Second malignant neoplasms and cardiovascular disease following radiotherapy. J Natl Cancer Inst. 2012;104(5):357–70. Epub

2012 Feb 6. PMID: 22312134; PMCID: PMC3295744. https://doi.org/10.1093/jnci/djr533.

3. Giordano SH, Kuo YF, Freeman JL, Buchholz TA, Hortobagyi GN, Goodwin JS. Risk of cardiac death after adjuvant radiotherapy for breast cancer. J Natl Cancer Inst. 2005;97(6):419–24. PMID: 15770005; PMCID: PMC1853253. https://doi.org/10.1093/jnci/dji067.

4. Plana JC, Galderisi M, Barac A, Ewer MS, Ky B, Scherrer-Crosbie M, et al. Expert consensus for multimodality imaging evaluation of adult patients during and after cancer therapy: a report from the American Society of Echocardiography and the European Association of Cardiovascular Imaging. Eur Heart J Cardiovasc Imaging. 2014;15(10):1063–93. PMID: 25239940; PMCID: PMC4402366. https://doi.org/10.1093/ehjci/jeu192.

5. Lancellotti P, Nkomo VT, Badano LP, Bergler-Klein J, Bogaert J, Davin L, et al. European Society of Cardiology Working Groups on Nuclear Cardiology and Cardiac Computed Tomography and Cardiovascular Magnetic Resonance; American Society of Nuclear Cardiology; Society for Cardiovascular Magnetic Resonance; Society of Cardiovascular Computed Tomography. Expert consensus for multi-modality imaging evaluation of cardiovascular complications of radiotherapy in adults: a report from the European Association of Cardiovascular Imaging and the American Society of Echocardiography. Eur Heart J Cardiovasc Imaging. 2013;14(8):721–40. Erratum in: Eur Heart J Cardiovasc Imaging. 2013 Dec;14(12):1217. PMID: 23847385. https://doi.org/10.1093/ehjci/jet123.

6. Desai MY, Wu M, Masri A, et al. Increased aorto-mitral curtain thickness independently predicts mortality in patients with radiation-associated cardiac disease undergoing cardiac surgery. Ann Thorac Surg. 2014;97:1348–55.

7. Reed GW, Masri A, Griffin BP, Kapadia SR, Ellis SG, Desai MY. Long-term mortality in patients with radiation-associated coronary artery disease treated with percutaneous coronary intervention. Circ Cardiovasc Interv. 2016;9

8. Donnellan E, Masri A, Johnston DR, et al. Long-term outcomes of patients with mediastinal radiation-associated severe aortic stenosis and subsequent surgical aortic valve replacement: a matched cohort study. J Am Heart Assoc. 2017;6

9. Darby SC, Ewertz M, McGale P, et al. Risk of ischemic heart disease in women after radiotherapy for breast cancer. N Engl J Med. 2013;368:987–98.

Chapter 15
Acute Coronary Syndrome in a Patient with Lung Cancer 2 Days After Second Cycle of Carboplatin and Paclitaxel

Clinical Case

Patient was a 62 years old female with stage IIB, T2 N1 non-small cell carcinoma/adenocarcinoma of the lung, treated with left lower lobectomy and started on adjuvant carboplatin and paclitaxel chemotherapy. The patient's past medical history includes hearing loss and bleeding peptic ulcer. Two days after starting chemotherapy, she felt very unwell with nausea, vomiting, fatigue, shortness of breath with exertion, and left-sided sharp, stabbing chest pain. She vomited multiple times.

On presentation to Emergency Room, patient was tachycardic, her heart rate was 106 bpm, regular, blood pressure 125/94 mmHg, respiratory rate 18 per minute and temperature 35.7 °C. Her oxygen saturation on room air was 100%. Blood work revealed hemoglobin 94 g/l, platelet count 60,000 per liter, potassium 2.6 mmol/l, sodium 127 mmol/l. Troponin I was 0.329 ng/ml (normal: less than 0.012).

© The Author(s), under exclusive license to Springer Nature Switzerland AG 2021
A. Rohani, *Clinical Cases in Cardio-Oncology*, Clinical Cases in Cardiology, https://doi.org/10.1007/978-3-030-71155-9_15

The patient was given Intra Venous (IV) normal saline. She was given oral potassium chloride 80 mEq as well as metoclopramide 10 mg IV.

Her ECG showed normal sinus rhythm with ST and T-wave abnormality. The patient's repeated troponin level were 0.319, (cut off point <0.012 ng/ml) she was provided with aspirin 81 mg daily, loading dose of 300 mg of clopido-grel and then 75 mg daily, enoxaparin 1 mg/kg every 12 hours, metoprolol 12.5 mg twice daily and rosuvastatin 20 mg daily.

Repeated blood work revealed potassium of 4.6 mmol/l and sodium 132 mEq/l.

The patient had chemotherapy induced emesis with hypo-kalemia, as a precipitating factor for non-ST elevation myo-cardial infarction (NSTEMI).

There are also case reports of paclitaxel induced acute coronary syndrome (ACS). In less than 4% of patients receiv-ing this drug, ACS can occur with unknown mechanism. This might have contributed to the presentation of NSTEMI in this patient as well.

There was discussion over the best plan of care in this case. It was decided to proceed with coronary angiogram despite moderate thrombocytopenia and employment of bare metal stent in case of need for PCI.

She underwent PCI to the LAD and RCA with bare metal stents and discharged home in stable clinical condition. Her platelet count was closely monitored and at this time there is no bleeding complications. She received dual antiplatelet therapy (DAPT) for 4 weeks and then continued with aspirin only. She was not started on chemotherapy again and is on observation plan for now.

Clinical Pearls

- On two trials (LEADERS FREE trial, Zotarolimus-Eluting Endeavor Sprint Stent in Uncertain DES Candidates—ZEUS trial) it was shown that second generation drug-eluting stents are preferable to bare-metal in the context of thrombocytopenia [1, 2].

- Avoidance of Nonsteroidal anti-inflammatory drugs (NSAIDs) suggested in the context of thrombocytopenia [3].
- A proton pump inhibitor can be considered along with DAPT for protection against GI bleeding [3].
- Radial approach for PCI is preferred [4].
- Prasugrel, ticagrelor and glycoprotein IIb/IIIa inhibitors should not be used in patients with thrombocytopenia [4].
- Platelet transfusion should be considered in patients who develop bleeding during or after cardiac catheterization [4].
- Table 15.1 summarizes the best antiplatelet treatment in the context of thrombocytopenia and ACS.
- Paclitaxel can cause cardiovascular toxicities including myocardial infarction with an incidence of 0.2–4% with an unknown exact mechanism. Both vasoconstriction (spasm) and direct thrombus formation, have been described in literature as a possible mechanism of ACS in patients receiving Paclitaxel [5–9].

TABLE 15.1 Thrombocytopenia and antiplatelet therapy

Platelet count	Plan for cardiac cath/PCI	Platelet treatment
10,000 < platelet < 30,000	Not recommended	Aspirin, needs risk/benefit analysis
30,000 < platelets < 50,000	Balloon angioplasty only	2 weeks DAPT – ACT should be monitored
Platelet > 50,000	Bare-metal stent (BMS)	4 weeks DAPT
	2nd or 3rd generation drug-eluting stents (DES)	6 months if optimal stent expansion was confirmed by IVUS or OCT.

OCT optical coherence tomography, *IVUS* intravascular ultrasound, *ACT* activated clotting time

- Cardiac arrhythmia is also observed in patients receiving paclitaxel [9, 10].

References

1. Valgimigli M, Patialiakas A, Thury A, McFadden E, Colangelo S, Campo G, et al. Zotarolimus-eluting versus bare-metal stents in uncertain drug-eluting stent candidates. J Am Coll Cardiol. 2015;65(8):805–15.
2. https://clinicaltrials.gov/ct2/show/NCT03118895
3. Long M, Ye Z, Zheng J, et al. Dual anti-platelet therapy following percutaneous coronary intervention in a population of patients with thrombocytopenia at baseline: a meta-analysis. BMC Pharmacol Toxicol. 2020;21:31.
4. McCarthy CP, Steg G, Bhatt DL. The management of antiplatelet therapy in acute coronary syndrome patients with thrombocytopenia: a clinical conundrum. Eur Heart J. 2017;38(47):3488.
5. Lluch A, Ojeda B, Colomer R, et al. Doxorubicin and paclitaxel in advanced breast carcinoma: importance of prior adjuvant anthracycline therapy. Cancer. 2000;89(11):2169–75. https://doi.org/10.1002/1097-0142(20001201)89:11<2169::aid-cncr4>3.0.co;2-9.
6. Giordano SH, Booser DJ, Murray JL, et al. A detailed evaluation of cardiac toxicity: a phase II study of doxorubicin and one- or three-hour-infusion paclitaxel in patients with metastatic breast cancer. Clin Cancer Res. 2002;8(11):3360–8.
7. Creager MA. Results of the CAPRIE trial: efficacy and safety of clopidogrel. Clopidogrel versus aspirin in patients at risk of ischaemic events. Vasc Med. 1998;3(3):257–60. https://doi.org/10.1177/1358836X9800300314.
8. Urban P, Meredith IT, Abizaid A, et al. Polymer-free drug-coated coronary stents in patients at high bleeding risk. N Engl J Med. 2015;373:2038–47.
9. Arbuck SG, Strauss H, Rowinsky E, et al. A reassessment of cardiac toxicity associated with Taxol. J Natl Cancer Inst Monogr. 1993;15:117–30.
10. Herrmann J, Yang EH, Iliescu CA, Cilingiroglu M, Charitakis K, Hakeem A, et al. Vascular toxicities of cancer therapies: the old and the new – an evolving avenue. Circulation. 2016;133:1272–89.

Chapter 16
Ibrutinib and Cardiac Arrythmias

Clinical Case

Patient was a 60-year-old male presented with palpitation. He denied chest pain, shortness of breath or syncope. He had background history of diabetes type 2, obstructive sleep apnea on CPAP and hypertension.

He was diagnosed with Primary central nervous system diffuse large B cell lymphoma 2 years ago. He received high-dose methotrexate, radiotherapy and currently on treatment with Ibrutinib 560 mg.

Physical examination was unremarkable except for irregularly irregular heartbeats.

ECG showed atrial fibrillation and PVCs with heart rate of 66 bpm.

He had normal myocardial perfusion scan. Echocardiogram showed normal LV size and systolic function, ejection fraction 55% and no hemodynamically significant valve disease, his left atrium volume index was normal. Patient was started on amiodarone and underwent successful electrical cardioversion with first attempt of 110 Joules and remained in normal sinus rhythm with small dose of bisoprolol. Amiodarone then stopped due to drug interactions with ibrutinib.

© The Author(s), under exclusive license to Springer Nature Switzerland AG 2021
A. Rohani, *Clinical Cases in Cardio-Oncology*, Clinical Cases in Cardiology, https://doi.org/10.1007/978-3-030-71155-9_16

Clinical Pearls

- Cardiac arrhythmias have occurred with Ibrutinib (tyrosine kinase inhibitor) therapy. The most frequent arrythmia is atrial fibrillation especially during the first 6 months of ibrutinib treatment, with the incidence of 3.3 per 100 person years. Life threatening arrhythmia like as ventricular tachycardia and ventricular fibrillation, was also reported; with a median time to onset of arrhythmia of 65 days from ibrutinib initiation [1].
- Age over 65 years, male gender, hypertension and previous history of AF, are risk factors for developing atrial fibrillation with Ibrutinib therapy [1].
- The benefit of ibrutinib treatment needs to be evaluated against the risk of arrythmia. Based on ibrutinib FDA tag, it needs to be stopped for any cardiac toxicity of grade 3 or greater. Once arrythmia resolved or back to grade 1, ibrutinib may be restarted again at the baseline dose. Dose reduction or discontinuation should be considered for refractory arrhythmias [2–4].

(For any arrythmia, grade 3 of toxicity means: symptomatic and uncontrolled arrythmia despite medical treatment, or controlled with a device; grade 4 is life-threatening arrhythmia associated with congestive heart failure, hypotension, syncope, shock and grade 5 of toxicity means: death.)

- Patient needs to be on anticoagulation based on CHADS65 Score [4].
- Ibrutinib has Moderate interaction with Factor Xa inhibitor (rivaroxaban, apixaban, edoxaban), these medications need to be used with caution, there is major interaction with Dabigatran. If creatinine clearance is normal, low molecular weight heparin can be considered as it was used in some clinical trials. Warfarin is an alternative with close INR monitoring [5, 6].
- Hypertension has also been reported with ibrutinib therapy [7].

- Ibrutinib-treated patients had higher risks of bleeding [5, 6].
- There are significant drug interactions between Ibrutinib, calcium channel blocker and amiodarone. The most appropriate choice for heart rate control is betablocker as there is less interaction. Having said that, carvedilol and nadolol might increase plasma concentrations of ibrutinib. Amiodarone also raises the serum concentration of ibrutinib by six- to ninefold [8, 9].
- There is less interaction between Class IB and IC antiarrhythmics with ibrutinib [10].
- Rate control strategy is preferred over rhythm control strategy, as there is high recurrence rate after cardioversion if patient still needs to be on ibrutinib.
- Ibrutinib may increase serum concentration of Digoxin. Digoxin should be taken at least 6 hours before or after taking ibrutinib to avoid toxic levels in the plasma.
- Calcium channel blockers like as diltiazem and verapamil increase ibrutinib serum concentration [10–12].

References

1. Leong DP, Caron F, Hillis C, et al. The risk of atrial fibrillation with ibrutinib use: a systematic review and meta-analysis. Blood. 2016;128:138–40.
2. Lampson BL, Yu L, Glynn RJ, et al. Ventricular arrhythmias and sudden death in patients taking ibrutinib. Blood. 2017;129:2581–4.
3. Ganatra S, Sharma A, Shah S, Chaudhry GM, Martin DT, Neilan TG, et al. Ibrutinib-associated atrial fibrillation. JACC Clin Electrophysiol. 2018;4(12):1491–500.
4. Brown JR, Moslehi J, O'Brien S, et al. Characterization of atrial fibrillation adverse events reported in ibrutinib randomized controlled registration trials. Haematologica. 2017;102:1796–805.
5. https://www.ccs.ca/images/Guidelines/Guidelines_POS_Library/2018%20AF%20Update_Supplement_Final.pdf
6. Yun S, Vincelette ND, Acharya U, Abraham I. Risk of atrial fibrillation and bleeding diathesis associated with ibrutinib treatment: a systematic review and pooled analysis of four

randomized controlled trials. Clin Lymphoma Myeloma Leuk. 2017;17:31–37.e13.

7. Caron F, Leong DP, Hillis C, Fraser G, Siegal D. Current understanding of bleeding with ibrutinib use: a systematic review and meta-analysis. Blood Adv. 2017;1:772–8.

8. Lee HJ, Chihara D, Wang M, Mouhayar E, Kim P. Ibrutinib-related atrial fibrillation in patients with mantle cell lymphoma. Leuk Lymphoma. 2016;57:2914–6.

9. IMBRUVICA Prescribing Information (www.imbruvica.com). January 2019. https://www.imbruvica.com/files/prescribing-information.pdf. Accessed 12 Dec 2019.

10. Shanafelt TD, Parikh SA, Noseworthy PA, et al. Atrial fibrillation in patients with chronic lymphocytic leukemia (CLL). Leuk Lymphoma. 2017;58:1630–9.

11. Levade M, David E, Garcia C, et al. Ibrutinib treatment affects collagen and von Willebrand factor-dependent platelet functions. Blood. 2014;124:3991–5.

12. Madgula AS, Singh M, Almnajam M, Pickett CC, Kim AS. Ventricular tachycardia storm in a patient treated with ibrutinib for waldenstrom macroglobulinemia. J Am Coll Cardiol CardioOncol. 2020;2(3):523–6.

Chapter 17
Dual Therapy BRAF Inhibitor Chemotherapy (Dabrafenib + Trametinib Chemotherapy) Induced Peripheral Edema

Clinical Case

Patient was an 83-year-old man with a history of melanoma of the right upper calf, positive BRAF mutation, he underwent surgical incision followed by chemotherapy with dabrafenib and Trametinib. Past medical history was significant for hypertension and dyslipidemia, well controlled on medications.

He was treated with combination of dabrafenib and trametinib for approximately 1 year. He developed bilateral 2+ peripheral edema. He was started on Lasix 40 mg and edema subsided. Subsequently he developed skin rash, a common side effect of dual therapy with dabrafenib and Trametinib chemotherapy.

Skin rash subsided with holding chemotherapy however both medications were restarted because of the appearance of suspicious lymph node on chest CT scan. He again developed skin rash (after 16th cycle of treatment). This time it was more generalized and associated with significant skin pruritus.

© The Author(s), under exclusive license to Springer Nature Switzerland AG 2021
A. Rohani, *Clinical Cases in Cardio-Oncology*, Clinical Cases in Cardiology, https://doi.org/10.1007/978-3-030-71155-9_17

He had contacted Oncology Service and was advised to discontinue both medications and present to Emergency Department.

On arrival to the Emergency Department, he was hemodynamically stable, heart rate 63 beats per minute, regular, blood pressure 104/75 mmHg, respiratory 20 per minute, and O_2 saturation 100% on room air. His body weight was 53 kg. His skin colour was normal, he has generalized fading urticarial rash covering his upper and lower extremities (grade 3 skin toxicity). JVP was flat. Carotid upstroke was brisk bilaterally. Heart sounds S1 and S2 were normal with systolic murmur grade 1/6 at left lower sternal border.

Chest auscultation revealed good air entry bilaterally, no adventitious sounds. Abdominal exam was unremarkable. He had 1+ ankle swelling bilaterally.

White blood cells 4.7/l, hemoglobin 103/l, platelets 228,000/l. Sodium 139 mmol/l, potassium 4.5 mmol/l, creatinine 61 mmol/l and GFR 81. Troponin negative.

For generalized urticaria rash, he was given Intravenous (IV) Benadryl 50 mg, IV ranitidine 50 mg and Methylprednisolone 125 mg IV.

Shortly after, he developed atrial fibrillation with rapid ventricular response, with heart rate of 165 beats per minute, his blood pressure remained stable.

This episode of AF could be just a coincidence, or the effect of cancer, inflammation, chemotherapy in the context of left atrial enlargement.

He was given bolus of fluid 500 cc, then IV amiodarone 150 mg with no response. Then after he was cardioverted successfully with synchronized 200 Joules shock. Post cardioversion, ECG showed normal sinus rhythm with isolated PACs, heart rate of 94 beats per minute and low voltage ECG as well as nonspecific ST/T abnormalities.

He was observed in the Emergency Department for several hours, remained hemodynamically stable and overall comfortable, his skin rash subsided.

He underwent regular stress test, reached target heart rate, with no evidence of ischemia.

He was started on apixaban 2.5 mg twice daily, as he was 55 kg and 83 years old. Most recent CT scan showed overall interval stability, without evidence of disease recurrence or disease progression.

Clinical Pearls

- Adverse reactions with dual therapy (trametinib plus dabrafenib) are as follows [1–5]:
- Hypertension.
- Peripheral edema,
- Heart failure with drop in LVEF.
- If there is asymptomatic drop in LVEF more than 10% and less than 20% from baseline, dual therapy needs to put on hold for 4 weeks. If LVEF improves to normal, it can be again re-started at a lower dose. After two dose reductions, if LVEF does not improved, it needs to be stopped permanently.
- In case of symptomatic HF or if LVEF dropped more than 20% from baseline, dual therapy must be stopped permanently.
- QTc prolongation: ECG and electrolytes should be checked before starting treatment, after 1 month of treatment and after any dose modifications.

Table 17.1 summarizes the best strategy for QT prolongation in patients on treatment with dual BRAF inhibitor chemotherapy. If baseline QTc is more than 500 ms, dual BRAF inhibitor chemotherapy should not be commenced.

TABLE 17.1 Strategy for QT prolongation in patients under treatment with Dual BRAF inhibitor chemotherapy

	QTc > 500 ms	>60 ms change from baseline
Discontinue permanently	+	+
Interrupt treatment until change in QTc < 60 ms from baseline and start at lower dose	–	+

References

1. Welsh SJ, Corrie PG. Management of BRAF and MEK inhibitor toxicities in patients with metastatic melanoma. Ther Adv Med Oncol. 2015;7(2):122–36. https://doi.org/10.1177/1758834014566428.
2. Flaherty K, Infante J, Daud A, Gonzalez R, Kefford R, Sosman J, et al. Combined BRAF and MEK inhibition in melanoma with BRAF V600 mutations. N Engl J Med. 2012a;367:1694–703.
3. Bronte E, Bronte G, Novo G, et al. Cardiotoxicity mechanisms of the combination of BRAF-inhibitors and MEK-inhibitors. Pharmacol Ther. 2018;192:65–73. https://doi.org/10.1016/j.pharmthera.2018.06.017.
4. Livingstone E, Zimmer L, Vaubel J, Schadendorf D. BRAF, MEK and KIT inhibitors for melanoma: adverse events and their management. Chin Clin Oncol. 2014;3(3):29.
5. Welsh SJ, Corrie PG. Management of BRAF and MEK inhibitor toxicities in patients with metastatic melanoma. Ther Adv Med Oncol. 2015;7(2):122–36.

Chapter 18
Vascular Endothelial Growth Factor (VEGF) Bevacizumab and Hypertension

Clinical Case

A 56-year-old male known for rectosigmoid cancer with peritoneal carcinomatosis, on FOLFIRI chemotherapy plus bevacizumab referred to cardio-oncology clinic for hypertension. He denied any cardiovascular related symptoms or history of hypertension in the past. He never smoked and was a nondrinker. On examination he had blood pressure 170/100 mmHg. His body mass index was 25 kg/m². Otherwise physical examination was unremarkable. A 12-lead electrocardiogram showed normal sinus rhythm with normal axis and heart rate of 75 bpm.

Echocardiogram revealed normal left ventricular size, systolic function, with no regional wall motion abnormalities, mild left ventricular hypertrophy. Grade I/IV diastolic dysfunction (abnormal relaxation filling pattern) and normal filling pressures. Global longitudinal strain (average) = −20%. Left ventricular ejection fraction was estimated at 66.4%.

He was started on ramipril, 5 mg/day, and blood pressure Holter monitor was ordered. It showed average daytime blood pressure of 165/100 mmHg. Dose of ramipril increased to 10 mg. On further follow up, his blood pressure still was not

© The Author(s), under exclusive license to Springer Nature Switzerland AG 2021
A. Rohani, *Clinical Cases in Cardio-Oncology*, Clinical Cases in Cardiology, https://doi.org/10.1007/978-3-030-71155-9_18

well controlled and was around 150/90 mmHg. He was started on combination of chlorthalidone 25 mg/day and amlodipine 10 mg/day. After this, he had marginal improvement in his blood pressure. FOLFIRI with bevacizumab, stopped due to evidence of progression of cancer on CT scan. He was then switched to third-line single agent panitumumab for eight cycles, unfortunately despite this, his cancer progressed and complicated by interactable ascites. He wished to hold off on radiotherapy and chemotherapy and plan for palliative care. His blood pressure was back to his baseline and all blood pressure medications stopped.

Clinical Pearls [1–3]

- Incidence of bevacizumab induced HTN is between 19% and 42%.
- Bevacizumab needs to put on hold if:

  - Blood pressure remains uncontrolled.
  - Hypertensive crisis or hypertensive encephalopathy happened.

- Frequent Monitoring of blood pressure in the first weeks of therapy suggested.
- Blood pressure Goal of 130/80 mmHg is considered acceptable for most of the patients.
- Definition of bevacizumab induced HTN is new onset increases in blood pressure ≥140/90 mmHg over the course of treatment or 20 mm increase in diastolic blood pressure from the baseline.
- High risk population for anti-VEGF (Vascular endothelial growth factor) therapy induced HTN include Preexisting hypertension, age ≥60 years, and body mass index (BMI) ≥25 kg/m^2
- In one study shorter bevacizumab infusions (0.5 mg/kg/min) associated with less risk of proteinuria and hypertension [3].

References

1. Mir O, Coriat R, Cabanes L, et al. An observational study of bevacizumab-induced hypertension as a clinical biomarker of antitumor activity. Oncologist. 2011;16(9):1325–32. https://doi.org/10.1634/theoncologist.2010-0002.
2. Sica DA. Angiogenesis inhibitors and hypertension: an emerging issue. J Clin Oncol. 2006;24(9):1329–31. https://doi.org/10.1200/JCO.2005.04.5740.
3. Shah SR, Gressett Ussery SM, Dowell JE, et al. Shorter bevacizumab infusions do not increase the incidence of proteinuria and hypertension. Ann Oncol. 2013;24(4):960–5. https://doi.org/10.1093/annonc/mds593.

Chapter 19
Amyloid Heart Disease

Clinical Case

The patient was a 65-year-old gentleman who was referred to cardiology service because of progressive shortness of breath on exertion, postural dizziness and an elevated BNP of 5450 ng/l. He had NYHA class 2. He denied chest pain, palpitation, orthopnea, PND, or syncope.

Chronology of symptoms:
He was diagnosed with an extensive unprovoked right leg deep vein thrombosis last year and started on Rivaroxaban 20 mg daily.

He subsequently developed bilateral lower extremity edema and was found to have nephrotic-range proteinuria with a 24-hour urine showing more than 3 g of protein. Then after patient developed progressive renal insufficiency and underwent renal biopsy which reported amyloidosis with 5/29 glomeruli globally sclerosed with mild interstitial fibrosis and tubular atrophy.

He has had intermittent drenching night sweats 2–3 times per week. There was no history of abnormal bruising, bleeding or skin changes. He has had progressive paresthesia involving his feet bilaterally.

© The Author(s), under exclusive license to Springer Nature Switzerland AG 2021
A. Rohani, *Clinical Cases in Cardio-Oncology*, Clinical Cases in Cardiology, https://doi.org/10.1007/978-3-030-71155-9_19

He underwent a bone marrow aspiration and biopsy which reported as lambda light chain restricted plasma cell neoplasm with 10% of cellularity in an interstitial distribution. Amyloid was noted in the bone marrow vessels. He was diagnosed with systemic AL amyloid disease. On examination, blood pressure 81/52 mmHg, pulse rate of 87 bpm, afebrile, oxygen saturation of 98% on room air. Chest was clear. No adventitious sound. Heart had normal S1, S2, with no murmur. Both lower extremities were symmetric in size with no edema.

He had an ECG, which showed sinus rhythm with first-degree AV block, PACs, left axis deviation, Q in the inferior leads, PR interval 210 ms, QT interval 490 ms, and bifascicular block.

WBC 5500/l, hemoglobin 126/l, platelet count 191,000/l. Sodium 131 mmol/l, potassium 4.2 mmol/l, creatinine 147 μmol/l, GFR 42 cc/min/1.73 m^2. First troponin 0.161 ng/cc. Last troponin 0.101 ng/cc, cut off point 0.034 ng/l. BNP 5450 ng/l, (disproportionately high, as patient was euvolemic on exam) cut off point 250 ng/l.

Chest x-ray was normal. coronary angiogram, showed distal Left Main disease, less than 10% stenosis, mild RCA disease, and mid focal 60% LAD stenosis.

He underwent an echocardiogram, which showed LVEF 39%, increased biventricular wall thickness, cardiac valve thickness and relative apical sparing on GLS (Figs. 19.1 and 19.2). He also underwent cardiac MRI which showed mild to moderate late Gadolinium enhancement related to cardiac amyloidosis. Patient diagnosed with score 3 Mayo staging system for AL amyloidosis (Table 19.1) which means median survival of 5 months (Table 19.2) [1, 2].

He was not a good candidate for stem cell transplant, (SCT) as he had elevated troponin, elevated creatinine and blood pressure of 81 mmHg. (SCT eligible patients are patients with systolic blood pressure >90 mmHg, troponin T < 0.06 ng/ml and serum creatinine ≤150 mmol/l.) He was offered   cyclophosphamide-bortezomib-dexamethasone chemotherapy.

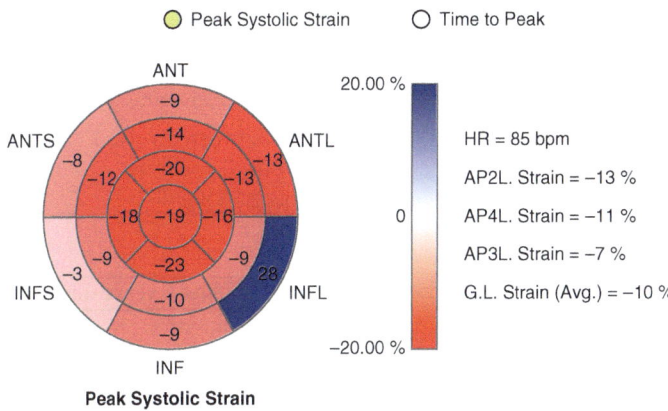

FIGURE 19.1 Relative apical sparing on longitudinal strain

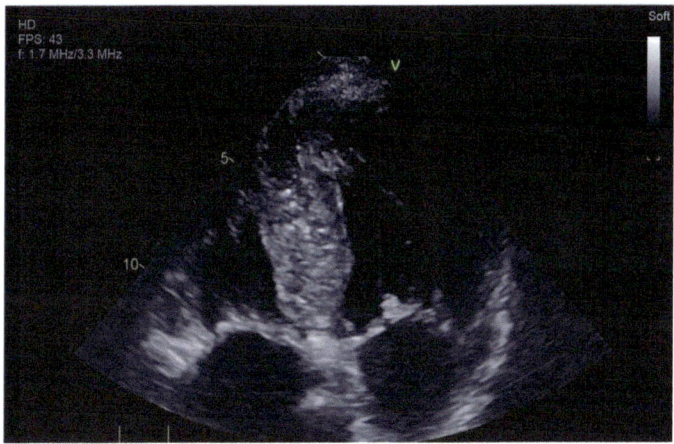

FIGURE 19.2 LVH on four chamber apical view, valvular thickness on TTE

TABLE 19.1 Mayo staging system for AL amyloidosis

	Score
NT-pro-BNP ≥ 1800 pg/ml	1
Troponin T ≥ 0.025 ng/ml	1
Difference between involved and uninvolved serum free light chains ≥ 18 mg/dl	1

TABLE 19.2 Median 5 years survival based on Mayo score

Score	Median 5 years survival
0	73 months
1	35 months
2	15 months
3	5 months

Clinical Pearls

- In patients with signs and symptoms of HF with one or more of the following features, amyloid heart disease should be considered as one of differential diagnosis [3]:
  - Unexplained Left ventricular hypertrophy;
  - Bilateral carpal tunnel syndrome;
  - Established AL (light chain) or ATTR (transthyretin) amyloidosis.
  - Nondiabetic nephrotic syndrome;
  - Hepatomegaly or increased alkaline phosphatase.
  - Peripheral sensorimotor neuropathy;
  - Weight loss, Unexplained fatigue, edema, or paresthesia in a patient with Monoclonal gammopathy.
  - Low flow–low gradient aortic valve stenosis in a patient older than 60 years old (commonly seen in patients with wild type ATTR Amyloidosis typically with preserved LVEF).

Relative apical sparing of global longitudinal strain (GLS) on TTE is a relatively specific finding in cardiac amyloidosis. Other infiltrative features on electrocardiogram (ECG) and echocardiogram include low QRS voltages on ECG despite LVH on echo, small pericardial effusion, and interatrial septal and valvular thickening.

- Natriuretic peptides could be quite high in patients with amyloidosis despite euvolemic presentation of patient.
- Treatment of cardiac amyloidosis [1, 2, 4, 5]:
  - For relief of congestion, loop diuretics and Aldosterone antagonist therapy (e.g., spironolactone) are the mainstay of treatment with close monitoring of blood pressure and renal function. Beta blockers and ACE inhibitors or angiotensin receptor blockers (ARBs) in patients with cardiac amyloidosis are poorly tolerated and there is no proven benefit from these group of medications.
  - Tafamidis can decrease the number of hospitalizations and deaths in patients with transthyretin (ATTR)-mediated amyloid cardiomyopathy and NYHA class I–III.
  - In AL amyloidosis chemotherapy with stem cell transplantation (SCT) are mainstay of treatment.
  - Patients with cardiac amyloidosis, particularly AL type are considered high risk for intracardiac thrombosis, and regardless of their CHADS2 or CHADS2-VA2SC score, in case of atrial fibrillation, they need to be anticoagulated with warfarin or one of direct oral anticoagulants (DOACs). Furthermore, anticoagulation should be considered even in a patient with normal sinus rhythm, AL type cardiac amyloidosis with low left atrial appendage emptying velocity on TEE or tiny trans mitral A wave on TTE [6].

References

1. Kumar S, Dispenzieri A, Lacy MQ, et al. Revised prognostic staging system for light chain amyloidosis incorporating cardiac biomarkers and serum free light chain measurements. J Clin Oncol. 2012;30(9):989–95. https://doi.org/10.1200/JCO.2011.38.5724.

2. Gertz MA. Immunoglobulin light chain amyloidosis: 2020 update on diagnosis, prognosis, and treatment. Am J Hematol. 2020;95(7):848–60. https://doi.org/10.1002/ajh.25819.
3. Maurer MS, Elliott P, Comenzo R, Semigran M, Rapezzi C. Addressing common questions encountered in the diagnosis and management of cardiac amyloidosis. Circulation. 2017;135(14):1357–77. https://doi.org/10.1161/CIRCULATIONAHA.116.024438.
4. Maurer MS, Schwartz JH, Gundapaneni B, et al. Tafamidis treatment for patients with transthyretin amyloid cardiomyopathy. N Engl J Med. 2018;379(11):1007–16. https://doi.org/10.1056/NEJMoa1805689.
5. Dispenzieri A, Katzmann JA, Kyle RA, Larson DR, Melton LJ III, Colby CL, Therneau TM, Clark R, Kumar SK, Bradwell A, Fonseca R, Jelinek DF, Rajkumar SV. Prevalence and risk of progression of light-chain monoclonal gammopathy of undetermined significance: a retrospective population-based cohort study. Lancet. 2010;375:1721–8.
6. Feng D, Syed IS, Martinez M, Oh JK, Jaffe AS, Grogan M, Edwards WD, Gertz MA, Klarich KW. Intracardiac thrombosis and anticoagulation therapy in cardiac amyloidosis. Circulation. 2009;119(18):2490–7. Epub 2009 May 4. PMID: 19414641. https://doi.org/10.1161/CIRCULATIONAHA.108.785014.

Chapter 20
Venous Thromboembolism in Cancer Patients

Clinical Pearls

- Risk of bleeding in cancer patients is higher than general population ranging from 6.5 to 18%; Table 20.1 summarizes safety of anticoagulation in the context of thrombocytopenia, which is quite common among cancer patients [1–3].
- Risk of thrombosis is significantly higher in multiple myeloma, acute leukemia, Gastric, brain and pancreatic cancer patients.
- Recurrent thrombosis in patients on anticoagulation, should prompt searching for occult malignancy.

Venous Thromboembolism Induced by Chemotherapy Drugs [4]

- Use of Tamoxifen in breast cancer patients is associated with an increased risk of VTE, with overall risk of 1–3% [5].
- Thromboembolic disease is common among patients with multiple myeloma on treatment with Revlimid plus high dose dexamethasone.

  - Treatment with Immunomodulatory drug (IMiD) such as thalidomide, lenalidomide, or pomalidomide in the

© The Author(s), under exclusive license to Springer Nature Switzerland AG 2021
A. Rohani, *Clinical Cases in Cardio-Oncology*, Clinical Cases in Cardiology, https://doi.org/10.1007/978-3-030-71155-9_20

TABLE 20.1 Primary VTE prophylaxis safety in the context of thrombocytopenia

Platelet counts above 50,000/μl	Safe
Platelet count is below the 20,000	Do not use anticoagulation
Above 20,000 but below 50,000 μl	Use anticoagulation if there is high-risk malignancy, (multiple myeloma, acute leukemia, Gastric, brain and pancreatic cancer.) or if there is history of previous thrombotic event.

context of multiple myeloma in combination with other agents (e.g., glucocorticoids, doxorubicin, or erythropoietin) could cause Thromboembolic events in greater than 20% of patients.

- The American Society of Clinical Oncology guidelines recommend thromboprophylaxis for patients receiving lenalidomide in combination with dexamethasone: aspirin for lower risk patients and low molecular weight heparin (LMWH) or therapeutic dose of warfarin for higher risk patients [4, 6–9].
- High risk patients include:

    Concomitant use of high dose dexamethasone (≥480 mg/month), doxorubicin, or multiagent chemotherapy.
    Presence of two or more risk factors (prior VTE, known inherited thrombophilia, central venous catheter or pacemaker, cardiac disease, DM, acute infection, use of erythropoietin, immobilization, obesity (BMI > 30 kg/m^2) and chronic kidney disease (GFR < 30)
    VTE prophylaxis (Table 20.1) is generally ordered if active therapy is continued.

- Lenalidomide may cause direct myocardial toxicity or exacerbate underlying myocardial dysfunction, patient must be cautioned about heart failure symptoms and need for a baseline echocardiogram.

- Increased incidence of VTE: in patients treated with cisplatin has been reported [10].
- Risk of DVT with ponatinib and bevacizumab also has been reported.

Catheter-Related Upper Extremity Venous Thrombosis [11–13]

Risk factors:

1. Prior DVT
2. Obesity
3. Recent surgery
4. Comorbidities like as diabetes and obstructive lung disease
5. Use of multi-lumen catheters
6. Mal-positioned catheters

Incidence: 5–15% in hospitalized patients and 2–5% in outpatient setting.

Treatment:

1. Removal of nonfunctional catheters in the context of DVT suggested, however in functioning catheters, removal is not recommended, as reinsertion is linked to higher risk of thrombosis.
2. Extremity elevation and nonsteroidal anti-inflammatory drugs [NSAIDs]for pain management.
3. Treatment with anticoagulation should be continued if catheter remains in place.
4. For isolated brachial vein thrombosis, individualized decision-making should be considered due to lack of evidence.

TABLE 20.2 Khorana score

Very high-risk type of cancer (stomach, pancreas)	2
High risk (lung, lymphoma, gynecologic, bladder, testicular)	1
Pre-chemotherapy platelet count ≥350,000/µl	1
Hemoglobin level <10 g/dl or use of ESAs	1
Pre-chemotherapy WBC >11,000/µl	1
BMI ≥ 35 kg/m^2	1

(a) A longer duration of anticoagulation may be warranted in a hospitalized patient with Khorana score (Table 20.2) of 2 or higher.

(b) Thrombolysis is indicated if there is:

- Severe symptoms despite anticoagulation.
- Thrombosis straddling both the subclavian and axillary veins.

Acute VTE in Patients with Brain Tumor

High Risk of Bleeding

1. Malignant primary tumors
2. Benign pituitary adenomas
3. Brain Metastases from melanoma, choriocarcinoma, thyroid carcinoma, and renal cell carcinoma
4. History of prior intracranial hemorrhage, or a remote history of a clinically significant intracranial hemorrhage.
5. Recent craniotomy
6. Treatment with Bevacizumab mostly in primary tumor

Treatment of acute VTE in patients with brain tumor:

- Decisions must be individualized: First it need to be proven that there is no evidence of acute intracranial hemorrhage on imaging and the potential benefits of anticoagulation outweigh the risk of bleeding.

Absolute contraindications of treatment:

- Acute (<48 hours) intracranial hemorrhage, (it is better to avoid anticoagulation in patients with remote history of a clinically significant intracranial hemorrhage or intratumoral hemorrhage within the past 4 weeks)
  - Uncontrolled malignant hypertension
  - Severe coagulopathy
  - Severe platelet dysfunction
  - Severe thrombocytopenia
  - Inherited bleeding disorder
  - High-risk invasive intracranial procedure within the last 7–14 days

Which Cancer Patients Needs VTE Prophylaxis

Inpatients:

Most hospitalized cancer patients with reduced mobility or patients undergoing surgery and are not at increased risk of bleeding, need thromboprophylaxis anticoagulation with low molecular weight (LMW) heparin, unfractionated heparin, or fondaparinux;

Outpatients:

Patients with higher baseline risk, like as Khorana (Table 20.2) score ≥ 2, multiple myeloma receiving an immunomodulatory drug (as mentioned above), pancreatic cancer with ONKOTEV score [14] (Table 20.3) of 2 or more needs anticoagulation. Direct factor Xa inhibitor such as apixaban (2.5 mg bid) or rivaroxaban (10 mg po daily) or a LMW heparin, at prophylactic dose can be considered. Table 20.4 summarizes agent of choice in specific cancer population.

TABLE 20.3 ONKOTEV score in pancreatic cancer

Presence of metastatic disease	1
Tumor compression of vascular/lymphatic structures	1
History of previous VTE (whether provoked or not)	1
Khorana score >2	1

TABLE 20.4 Agent selection for treatment of VTE in specific cancer population [15, 16, 17]

Brain tumor	LMW heparin
General	LMW heparin or apixaban
Renal insufficiency	Intravenous unfractionated heparin, warfarin
Pregnancy or pregnancy risk	LMW heparin
Coronary artery disease	Rivaroxaban, apixaban, edoxaban, Warfarin. Antiplatelet therapy should be avoided if possible
Liver disease	LMW heparin
GI bleeding	Apixaban

A recent Systematic Review and Meta-Analysis by Sabatino et al., demonstrated in patients with active cancer, direct oral anticoagulants are equivalent to LMWH in preventing VTE recurrence, however risk of nonmajor bleeding is increased with DOACs especially in patients with GI malignancy [15].

In another recent Randomized Controlled Trial, it was concluded that in patients with VTE and active cancer, Apixaban (10 mg twice daily for 7 days followed by 5 mg twice daily) is a suitable alternative to LMWH [16].

References

1. Sørensen HT, Mellemkjaer L, Olsen JH, Baron JA. Prognosis of cancers associated with venous thromboembolism. N Engl J Med. 2000;343(25):1846–50.
2. Carrier M, Abou-Nassar K, Mallick R, et al. Apixaban to prevent venous thromboembolism in patients with cancer. N Engl J Med. 2019;380(8):711–9.
3. Key NS, Khorana AA, Kuderer NM, et al. Venous thromboembolism prophylaxis and treatment in patients with cancer: ASCO clinical practice guideline update. J Clin Oncol. 2020;38(5):496–520.
4. Ramot Y, Nyska A, Spectre G. Drug-induced thrombosis: an update. Drug Saf. 2013;36(8):585–603.
5. Bushnell CD, Goldstein LB. Risk of ischemic stroke with tamoxifen treatment for breast cancer: a meta-analysis. Neurology. 2004;63(7):1230–3.
6. Larocca A, Cavallo F, Bringhen S, Di Raimondo F, Falanga A, Evangelista A, et al. Aspirin or enoxaparin thromboprophylaxis for patients with newly diagnosed multiple myeloma treated with lenalidomide. Blood. 2012;119(4):933–9.
7. Baz R, Li L, Kottke-Marchant K, et al. The role of aspirin in the prevention of thrombotic complications of thalidomide and anthracycline-based chemotherapy for multiple myeloma. Mayo Clin Proc. 2005;80(12):1568–74.
8. Ikhlaque N, Seshadri V, Kathula S, Baumann MA. Efficacy of prophylactic warfarin for prevention of thalidomide-related deep venous thrombosis. Am J Hematol. 2006;81(6):420–2. https://doi.org/10.1002/ajh.20625.
9. Zangari M, Barlogie B, Anaissie E, et al. Deep vein thrombosis in patients with multiple myeloma treated with thalidomide and chemotherapy: effects of prophylactic and therapeutic anticoagulation. Br J Haematol. 2004;126(5):715–21.
10. Moore RA, Adel N, Riedel E, et al. High incidence of thromboembolic events in patients treated with cisplatin-based chemotherapy: a large retrospective analysis. J Clin Oncol. 2011;29(25):3466–73.

11. Fallouh N, McGuirk HM, Flanders SA, Chopra V. Peripherally inserted central catheter-associated deep vein thrombosis: a narrative review. Am J Med. 2015;128(7):722–38.
12. Chopra V, Ratz D, Kuhn L, Lopus T, Lee A, Krein S. Peripherally inserted central catheter-related deep vein thrombosis: contemporary patterns and predictors. J Thromb Haemost. 2014;12(6):847–54.
13. Debourdeau P, Farge D, Beckers M, et al. International clinical practice guidelines for the treatment and prophylaxis of thrombosis associated with central venous catheters in patients with cancer. J Thromb Haemost. 2013;11(1):71–80.
14. Cella CA, Di Minno G, Carlomagno C, et al. Preventing venous thromboembolism in ambulatory cancer patients: the ONKOTEV study. Oncologist. 2017;22(5):601–8. https://doi.org/10.1634/theoncologist.2016-0246.
15. Sabatino J, De Osa S, Polimeni A, Sorrentino S, Indolfi C. Direct oral anticoagulants in patients with active cancer: a systematic review and meta-analysis. J Am Coll Cardiol CardioOncol. 2020;2(3):428–40.
16. Agnelli G, Becattini C, Meyer G, Muñoz A, Huisman MV, Connors JM, Cohen A, Bauersachs R, Brenner B, Torbicki A, Sueiro MR, Lambert C, Gussoni G, Campanini M, Fontanella A, Vescovo G, Verso M, Caravaggio Investigators. Apixaban for the treatment of venous thromboembolism associated with cancer. N Engl J Med. 2020;382(17):1599–607. Epub 2020 Mar 29. PMID: 32223112. https://doi.org/10.1056/NEJMoa1915103.
17. McBane RD II, Wysokinski WE, Le-Rademacher JG, et al. Apixaban and dalteparin in active malignancy-associated venous thromboembolism: the ADAM VTE trial. J Thromb Haemost. 2020;18(2):411–21. https://doi.org/10.1111/jth.14662.

Chapter 21
QT Prolongation in Cancer Patients

Clinical Pearls

- High risk chemotherapy drugs associated with Acquired long QT interval include: Arsenic trioxide, serotonin reuptake inhibitors (SRIs) concomitant with tamoxifen, tyrosine kinase inhibitors (imatinib, Dasatinib), vascular disruption agents, Capecitabine, oxaliptin, vandetanib, Pazopanib, cediranib and sunitinib [1–6].
- Romidepsin and Vorinostat (histone deacetylase inhibitors) which are indicated for treatment of Cutaneous T-cell lymphoma can also cause QT interval prolongation.
- There is also increased risk of long QT from supportive therapies such as ondansetron as well as concomitant antibiotic use like as macrolides and quinolons [7–9].
- Infection, anemia, hypothyroidism, Electrolyte disturbances are quite common in cancer patients and should be corrected promptly.
- Chronic proton pump inhibitor is also associated with long QT and could be the result of hypomagnesemia [10].
- Patients with acquired long QT interval would be at risk for developing life threatening torsade de pointes (TdP). Figure 21.1 shows TDP in a patient with hypokalemia (Fig. 21.2, shows ECG in normal sinus rhythm) which was treated promptly with cardioversion, replenishment of

© The Author(s), under exclusive license to Springer Nature Switzerland AG 2021
A. Rohani, *Clinical Cases in Cardio-Oncology*, Clinical Cases in Cardiology, https://doi.org/10.1007/978-3-030-71155-9_21

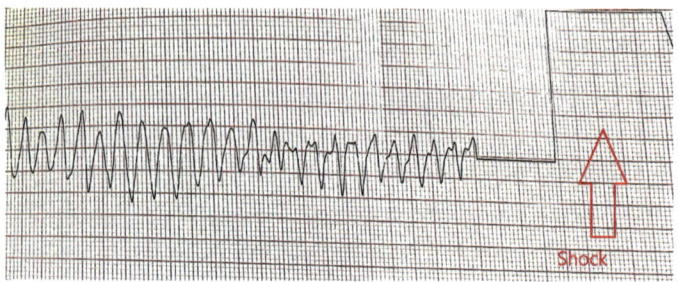

FIGURE 21.1 TDP in a patient with hypokalemia which was treated promptly with cardioversion

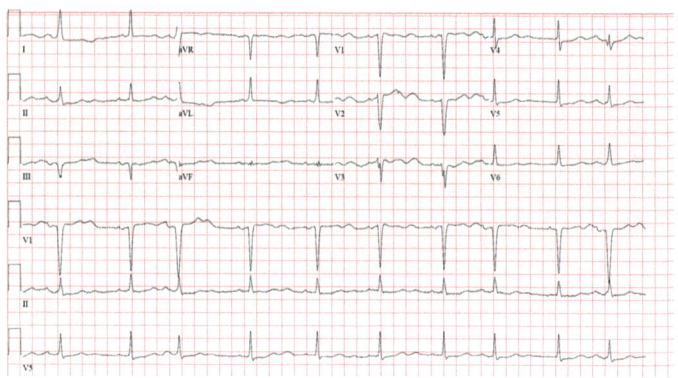

FIGURE 21.2 Hypokalemia and long QT

potassium, 2-g IV bolus of magnesium sulfate and intravenous isoproterenol 2 mcg/min to keep baseline heart rate around 100 bpm. Figure 21.2 shows same patient on arrival to hospital with aborted sudden cardiac death.

- Normal QTc interval is between 350 and 450 ms in adult men and between 360 and 460 ms in adult women.

- There are four formula for calculation of QT:

  - Bazett formula: $QT \div \sqrt{RR}$: This formula is most extensively employed, but overcorrects at fast heart rate (HR) and under-corrects at slower HR [9–11].
  - Fridericia formula: $QT/RR^{1/3}$, is used more frequently in oncology patients as it is more accurate at slower HR and establishes less overcorrection at faster HR [12].
  - Framingham formula: $QT + 0.154 (1 - RR)$
  - Hodges formula: $QT + 1.75$ (heart rate $- 60$). This one is using especially at Heart Rate >90 bpm

- When there is left bundle branch block, right bundle branch block, or paced rhythm, 48.5% of the duration of the QRS should be subtracted and then needs to be corrected for HR or simply QTc of >550 ms can be considered abnormal in this context.
- Best leads for QT measurement are leads II and V5 as these two show the earliest QRS onset and the latest end of the T wave.
- As a rule, an anticancer drug should be stopped if the QTc is >500 ms or QT interval prolonged more than 60 ms during treatment.
- Avoid citalopram, escitalopram and paroxetine in patients treated with tamoxifen. Venlafaxine and fluvoxamine have less risk.
- This website: https://www.crediblemeds.org can be used for drugs that can cause prolongation of QT interval.
- Table 21.1 shows QT interval monitoring frequency in three group of anticancer medications.

TABLE 21.1 QT interval monitoring frequency

Drug	ECG monitoring frequency	
Arsenic trioxide [4–6]	Baseline and weekly ECG	Spontaneously returns to baseline values after 8 weeks-hold therapy if the QT interval is greater than 500 ms. When the QT interval is below 460 ms, it can be restarted with careful monitoring of magnesium and potassium
Vandetanib	Baseline ECG, at 2–4 weeks and at 8–12 weeks after the start, and then every 3 months	
Nilotinib	If baseline ECG has QTc less than 480 ms repeat ECG in 3–6 months. If dose of Nilotinib increased, 3–5 days after dose adjustment, ECG should be repeated.	

References

1. Porta-Sánchez A, Gilbert C, Spears D, et al. Incidence, diagnosis, and management of QT prolongation induced by cancer therapies: a systematic review. J Am Heart Assoc. 2017;6(12):e007724.
2. Hussaarts KGAM, Berger FA, Binkhorst L, Oomen-de Hoop E, van Leeuwen RWF, van Alphen RJ, Mathijssen-van Stein D, de Groot NMS, Mathijssen RHJ, van Gelder T. The risk of QTc-interval prolongation in breast cancer patients treated with tamoxifen in combination with serotonin reuptake inhibitors. Pharm Res. 2019;37(1):7. PMID: 31845095; PMCID: PMC6914733. https://doi.org/10.1007/s11095-019-2746-9.

3. Goldsmith S, From AH. Arsenic-induced atypical ventricular tachycardia. N Engl J Med. 1980;303:1096–8.
4. Little RE, Kay GN, Cavender JB, et al. Torsade de pointes and T-U wave alternans associated with arsenic poisoning. Pacing Clin Electrophysiol. 1990;13:164–70.
5. St Petery J, Gross C, Victorica BE. Ventricular fibrillation caused by arsenic poisoning. Am J Dis Child. 1970;120:367–71.
6. Weinberg SL. The electrocardiogram in acute arsenic poisoning. Am Heart J. 1960;60:971–5.
7. Coppola C, Rienzo A, Piscopo G, Barbieri A, Arra C, Maurea N. Management of QT prolongation induced by anti-cancer drugs: target therapy and old agents. Different algorithms for different drugs. Cancer Treatment Rev. 2018:135–43.
8. Tamargo J, Caballero R, Delpon E. Cancer chemotherapy and cardiac arrhythmias: a review. Drug Saf. 2015;38:129–52.
9. Locatelli M, Criscitello C, Esposito A, et al. QTc prolongation induced by targeted biotherapies used in clinical practice and under investigation: a comprehensive review. Target Oncol. 2015;10:27–43.
10. Amularo G, Gasbarrone L, Minisola G. Hypomagnesemia and proton-pump inhibitors. Expert Opin Drug Saf. 2013;12:709–16.
11. Rabkin SW, Cheng XB. Nomenclature, categorization and usage of formulae to adjust QT interval for heart rate. World J Cardiol. 2015;7:315–25.
12. Borad MJ, Soman AD, Benjamin M, et al. Effect of selection of QTc formula on eligibility of cancer patients for phase I clinical trials. Invest New Drugs. 2013;31:1056–65.

Chapter 22
Cardiovascular Implantable Electronic Devices (CIEDs) in cancer Patients Needs Radiation Therapy

Clinical Case

A 71-year-old female, smoker, with a dual-chamber pacemaker, for symptomatic second-degree atrioventricular block presented with cough, wheezing and shortness of breath over the last 2 months. On examination intermittent wheezing noted. Covid 19 test was negative. Chest CT scan revealed a left lower lobe lung mass and one enlarged mediastinal lymph node measuring 1.9 cm.

Her baseline ECG showed normal sinus rhythm with heart rate of 64 bpm and bi-fascicular block: Right Bundle Branch Block and Left Anterior Fascicular Block (RBBB+LAFB)

Bronchoscopy with biopsy revealed stage III non-small cell lung cancer, believed to be unresectable. Given her other comorbidities, she was scheduled for Radiation therapy only: total dose of 66 Gy in 30 fractions (2.2 Gy/fraction). The dose of radiation which is being planned was way higher than the recommended dose by the pacemaker company.

She has not been dependent on pacemaker and most of the time she had her own heart rhythm. She has been paced less than 20% of the time and mostly the right atrium was

A. Rohani, *Clinical Cases in Cardio-Oncology*, Clinical Cases in Cardiology, https://doi.org/10.1007/978-3-030-71155-9_22

paced. According to the site of the target of radiation therapy, the pacemaker was directly in the way of radiation and deemed to be at medium risk for pacemaker complications.

She underwent ECG-monitoring during radiotherapy and weekly Pacemaker interrogation. She remained stable with no pacemaker issues.

Clinical Pearls

- Radiation therapy could cause oversensing, temporarily increase in pacing rates, device resets, early battery depletion and complete device failure [1].
- Table 22.1 summarizes a practical approach for patients with pacemakers, who need radiation treatment [1, 2].
- Implantable cardioverter-defibrillator (ICD) are more sensitive to radiotherapy. ICD should be inactivated during treatment sessions by application of a magnet or reprogramming. Patient's heart rhythm needs to be closely monitored as soon as antitachycardia therapies are switched off. ICD needs to be interrogated on a weekly basis [3, 4].
- Follow-up interrogation schedule after completion of radiotherapy should be arranged on 1-, 3- and 6-months post treatment [5].
- In patients with cancer with overall poor prognosis, (survival less than 1 year), ICD therapy is not recommended.

TABLE 22.1 Practical approach for patients with pacemakers, who need radiotherapy [6, 7]

Risk	Low	Medium		High
Radiation dose	<2 Gy	<2 Gy	2–10 Gy	>10 Gy
Pace dependent	No	Yes	No	Yes
Plan	Routine measures, audiovisual assessment of the patient during RT	Weekly interrogation ECG-monitoring during radiation—external pacing should be available		– Consider repositioning of pacemaker in pacemaker dependent patients with ipsilateral breast or lung cancer – ECG-monitoring during radiotherapy – Pacemaker interrogation within 24 hours of radiotherapy after each session

References

1. Hurkmans CW, Knegjens JL, Oei BS, et al. Management of radiation oncology patients with a pacemaker or ICD: a new comprehensive practical guideline in The Netherlands. Dutch Society of Radiotherapy and Oncology (NVRO). Radiat Oncol. 2012;7:198.
2. Marbach JR, Sontag MR, Van Dyk J, Wolbarst AB. Management of radiation oncology patients with implanted cardiac pacemakers: report of AAPM Task Group No. 34. American Association of Physicists in Medicine. Med Phys. 1994;21:85–90.
3. Lambert P, Da Costa A, Marcy PY, et al. Pacemaker, implanted cardiac defibrillator and irradiation: management proposal in

2010 depending on the type of cardiac stimulator and prognosis and location of cancer. Cancer Radiother. 2011;15:238–49.

4. Brambatti M, Mathew R, Strang B, et al. Management of patients with implantable cardioverter-defibrillators and pacemakers who require radiation therapy. Heart Rhythm. 2015;12:2148–54.

5. Zaremba T, Jakobsen AR, Søgaard M, Thøgersen AM, Riahi S. Radiotherapy in patients with pacemakers and implantable cardioverter defibrillators: a literature review. EP Europace. 2016;18(4):479–91.

6. Kesek M, Nyholm T, Asklund T. Radiotherapy and pacemaker: 80 Gy to target close to the device may be feasible. Europace. 2012;14:1595.

7. Makkar A, Prisciandaro J, Agarwal S, Lusk M, Horwood L, Moran J, et al. Effect of radiation therapy on permanent pacemaker and implantable cardioverter-defibrillator function. Heart Rhythm. 2012;9:1964–8.

Chapter 23
Atrial Fibrillation in Cancer Patients

Clinical Pearls

In all patients with nonvalvular atrial fibrillation, (AF) including patients with underlying cancer, there is need to investigate reversible causes of AF, like as hyperthyroidism, structural heart disease (ischemia, valvular heart disease) and sleep apnea.

After shared decision making with the patient, either rate control or rhythm control strategy should be arranged. For patients at younger age, (less than 65 years old) at least, one time of cardioversion should be tried.

Table 23.1 summarizes suitable candidates for rate versus rhythm control strategy. However, clinician needs to individualize this decision based on clinical findings and overall prognosis and goal of care for each patient [2, 3].

Lung Cancer

There is a high occurrence rate of atrial fibrillation, especially during surgery for lung cancer [1].

Predictors of post-operative AF:

© The Author(s), under exclusive license to Springer Nature Switzerland AG 2021
A. Rohani, *Clinical Cases in Cardio-Oncology*, Clinical Cases in Cardiology, https://doi.org/10.1007/978-3-030-71155-9_23

TABLE 23.1 Rate vs rhythm control strategy

Rate control	Rhythm control
Need for cancer treatment which triggers AF	Persistent symptoms
Asymptomatic patients	Poor rate control
Advanced cancer stage	Reversible etiology like as hyperthyroidism
Severely dilated left atrium size >48 cc/BSA	Young patients with overall good prognosis and no structural heart disease
Frailty	
Early recurrence of AF < 1 month after cardioversion	
Chemotherapy with Ponatinib, Zanubrutinib, Ibrutinib, Alemtuzumab	

BSA body surface area, *AF* atrial fibrillation

- Increase in BNP (brain natriuretic peptide) 24 hours before or 1 hour after surgery.
- Echocardiographic indexes which is indicative of high risk for atrial fibrillation include: left ventricular diastolic dysfunction or increased left ventricular diastolic pressures. A mitral E/e′ ratio >8 on Doppler echocardiogram was highly sensitive (90% sensitivity) for predicting postoperative AF.
- Advanced age
- Male sex
- Prolonged surgery
- Advanced stage of cancer
- Need for post-operative blood transfusion.
- History of hypertension

Anticoagulation

- There are two risk calculation scores:

  For assessment of risk of thrombosis:

1. CHA2DS2-VASc: [4] congestive heart failure, hypertension, age of 75 years and older, (2 points) diabetes mellitus, previous stroke or transient ischemic attack, vascular disease, (2 points) 65–74 years of age, (1 point) female sex

   For analysis of risk of bleeding:

2. HAS-BLED: [5] hypertension, abnormal renal/liver function, stroke, bleeding history or predisposition, labile international normalized ratio, elderly, drugs/alcohol concomitantly.

   However, these two risk calculators have not been validated in cancer patients.

- High bleeding risk population among cancer patients:
  - HAS-BLED risk of 3 or more
  - Intracranial tumor
  - Hematologic malignancies with coagulation defects
  - Cancer therapy-induced thrombocytopenia
  - Severe metastatic hepatic disease
  - Luminal gastrointestinal cancers

  In this high-risk population left atrium appendage (LAA) closure either percutaneous or by surgery should be considered. If patient can take anticoagulation for at least 45 days after procedure and there is no history of prior cardiac surgery, patient can be considered for percutaneous closure.

- There is drug interaction between apixaban and rivaroxaban with drugs that are Inhibitors of CYP3A4 (Strong) and P-glycoprotein like as Dasatinib, Ibrutinib, Zanubrutinib and Grapefruit juice. Patients need close monitoring for any signs or symptoms of bleeding.

References

1. Vaporciyan AA, Correa AM, Rice DC, et al. Risk factors associated with atrial fibrillation after noncardiac thoracic surgery: analysis of 2588 patients. J Thorac Cardiovasc Surg. 2004;127(3):779–86. https://doi.org/10.1016/j.jtcvs.2003.07.011.
2. Farmakis D, Parissis J, Filippatos G. Insights into onco-cardiology: atrial fibrillation in cancer. J Am Coll Cardiol. 2014;63(10):945–53. https://doi.org/10.1016/j.jacc.2013.11.026.
3. Delluc A, Wang T-F, Yap E-S, Ay C, Schaefer J, Carrier M, et al. Anticoagulation of cancer patients with non-valvular atrial fibrillation receiving chemotherapy: guidance from the SSC of the ISTH. J Thromb Haemost. 2019;17(8):1247–52.
4. Lip GY, Nieuwlaat R, Pisters R, Lane DA, Crijns HJ. Refining clinical risk stratification for predicting stroke and thromboembolism in atrial fibrillation using a novel risk factor-based approach: the euro heart survey on atrial fibrillation. Chest. 2010;137(2):263–72.
5. Pisters R, Lane DA, Nieuwlaat R, de Vos CB, Crijns HJ, Lip GY. A novel user-friendly score (HAS-BLED) to assess 1-year risk of major bleeding in patients with atrial fibrillation: the Euro Heart Survey. Chest. 2010;138(5):1093–100.

Chapter 24
Pericardial Disease in Cancer Patients

Clinical Pearls

Pericardial effusion (Fig. 24.1) in the context of malignant tumors, could cause by followings [1–5]:

1. Cancer treatment induced pericardial effusion: cyclophosphamide, cytarabine, bleomycin, fludarabine, doxorubicin, docetaxel, immune checkpoint inhibitors, Dasatinib and Radiation therapy.

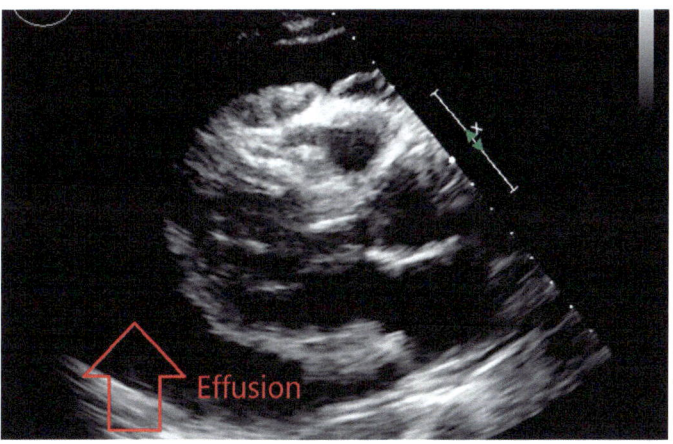

FIGURE 24.1 Pericardial effusion, para sternal long axis view TTE

© The Author(s), under exclusive license to Springer Nature Switzerland AG 2021
A. Rohani, *Clinical Cases in Cardio-Oncology*, Clinical Cases in Cardiology, https://doi.org/10.1007/978-3-030-71155-9_24

2. Malignant involvement of the pericardium: The most common tumor associated with pericardial disease, is lung cancer; others include breast, esophageal cancer, melanoma, lymphoma, and leukemia.
3. The first manifestation of cancer might be pericardial effusion and effusion can occur before cancer is evident. Because of this, especially in patients with malaise, weakness, unexplained weight loss with smoking history, if there is new large pericardial effusion or cardiac tamponade, a detailed investigation should be done to rule out underlying malignancy.
4. Presence of dyspnea, hypotension and tachycardia should raise the suspicion for clinical tamponade. Echocardiographic signs of tamponade include:

   (a) Presence of right ventricular diastolic collapse.
   (b) Right atrium systolic collapse.
   (c) Dilated inferior vena cava with no respiratory variation, (IVC congestion).
   (d) More than 25% Mitral inflow E velocity change with inspiration (decrease).
   (e) More than 40% Tricuspid inflow E velocity change with expiration.

5. Pericardial fluid should be sent for cytologic examination: The sensitivity of cytology for the diagnosis of a malignant effusion is between 67 and 92% [5–7].
6. Treatment of hemodynamically significant pericardial effusion is drainage. Echocardiographic guided pericardiocentesis can be done with the rate of major complications around 0.3–3.9%. The catheter should stay in the pericardial sac until drainage is <25 to 50 ml to none in a 24-hour period [8].
7. Presence of pericardial effusion affects the prognosis in cancer patients. Positive cytology for malignancy was an independent predictor of shortened survival in patients

with symptomatic malignant pericardial effusion with median survival of 2–4 months reported in observational studies [9].

8. Prevention of recurrence: Pericardial sclerosis or creation of a pericardial window by percutaneous balloon pericardiotomy or by surgery can reduce the recurrence rate [10].

References

1. DeCamp MM Jr, Mentzer SJ, Swanson SJ, Sugarbaker DJ. Malignant effusive disease of the pleura and pericardium. Chest. 1997;112(4 Suppl):291S–5S. https://doi.org/10.1378/chest.112.4_supplement.291s.

2. Maisch B, Ristic A, Pankuweit S. Evaluation and management of pericardial effusion in patients with neoplastic disease. Prog Cardiovasc Dis. 2010;53(2):157–63.

3. Klatt EC, Heitz DR. Cardiac metastases. Cancer. 1990;65(6):1456–9. https://doi.org/10.1002/1097-0142(19900315)65:6<1456:aid-cncr2820650634>3.0.co;2-5.

4. Gross JL, Younes RN, Deheinzelin D, Diniz AL, Silva RA, Haddad FJ. Surgical management of symptomatic pericardial effusion in patients with solid malignancies. Ann Surg Oncol. 2006;13(12):1732–8. https://doi.org/10.1245/s10434-006-9073-1.

5. Dequanter D, Lothaire P, Berghmans T, Sculier JP. Severe pericardial effusion in patients with concurrent malignancy: a retrospective analysis of prognostic factors influencing survival. Ann Surg Oncol. 2008;15(11):3268–71. https://doi.org/10.1245/s10434-008-0059-z.

6. Dosios T, Theakos N, Angouras D, Asimacopoulos P. Risk factors affecting the survival of patients with pericardial effusion submitted to subxiphoid pericardiostomy. Chest. 2003;124(1):242–6. https://doi.org/10.1378/chest.124.1.242.

7. Gornik HL, Gerhard-Herman M, Beckman JA. Abnormal cytology predicts poor prognosis in cancer patients with pericardial effusion. J Clin Oncol. 2005;23(22):5211–6. https://doi.org/10.1200/JCO.2005.00.745.

8. Tsang TS, Enriquez-Sarano M, Freeman WK, Barnes ME, Sinak LJ, Gersh BJ, Bailey KR, Seward JB. Consecutive 1127 therapeutic echocardiographically guided pericardiocenteses: clinical profile, practice patterns, and outcomes spanning 21 years. Mayo Clin Proc. 2002;77:429–36.

9. Akyuz S, Zengin A, Arugaslan E, Yazici S, Onuk T, Ceylan US, Gungor B, Gurkan U, Kemaloglu Oz T, Kasikcioglu H, Cam N. Echo-guided pericardiocentesis in patients with clinically significant pericardial effusion. Outcomes over a 10-year period. Herz. 2015;40 Suppl 2:153–9.

10. Puri A, Agarwal N, Dwivedi SK, Narain VS. Percutaneous balloon pericardiotomy for the treatment of recurrent malignant pericardial effusion. Indian Heart J. 2012;64(1):88–9. https://doi.org/10.1016/S0019-4832(12)60018-2.

Chapter 25
Large Cardiac Mass, an Incidental Finding in a Patient with Breast Cancer

Clinical Case

A 68 years old female post left mastectomy for invasive ductal carcinoma of right breast, scheduled for adjuvant chemotherapy. She denies any cardiovascular related symptoms. Her past medical history was significant for hypertension, gastric bypass surgery and Obstructive sleep apnea on CPAP. On examination she looks generally well, blood pressure 120/70, chest is clear. No adventitious sound, heart has normal S1, S2 with no murmur, both extremities are symmetric in size, with no edema. As part of a routine pre-chemotherapy screen, underwent an echocardiogram which revealed two large masses in her right atrium. The larger lesion measures about 7 × 4.5 cm, a smaller lesion is less than 2 cm in diameter (Figs. 25.1 and 25.2). First it considered to be a metastatic breast cancer lesion and the plan was follow up by echocardiogram, while chemotherapy progresses to see if there has been any change in size of masse with chemotherapy. She received four cycles of doxorubicin and cyclophosphamide followed by four cycles paclitaxel and adjuvant radiotherapy to right breast and regional lymph nodes.

© The Author(s), under exclusive license to Springer Nature Switzerland AG 2021
A. Rohani, *Clinical Cases in Cardio-Oncology*, Clinical Cases in Cardiology, https://doi.org/10.1007/978-3-030-71155-9_25

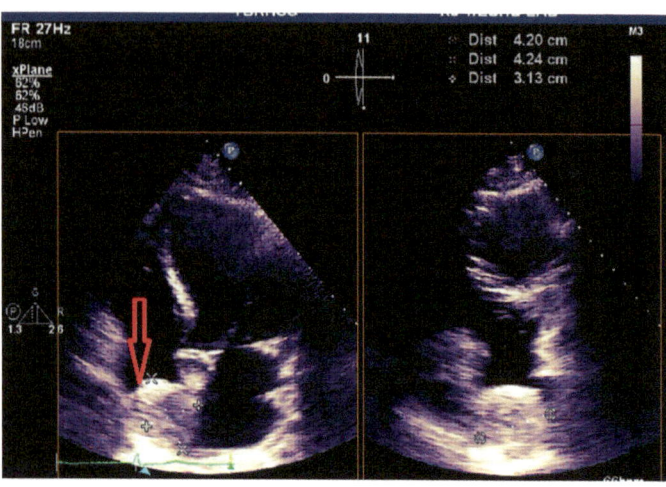

FIGURE 25.1 Apical four chamber TTE shows RA mass: red arrow

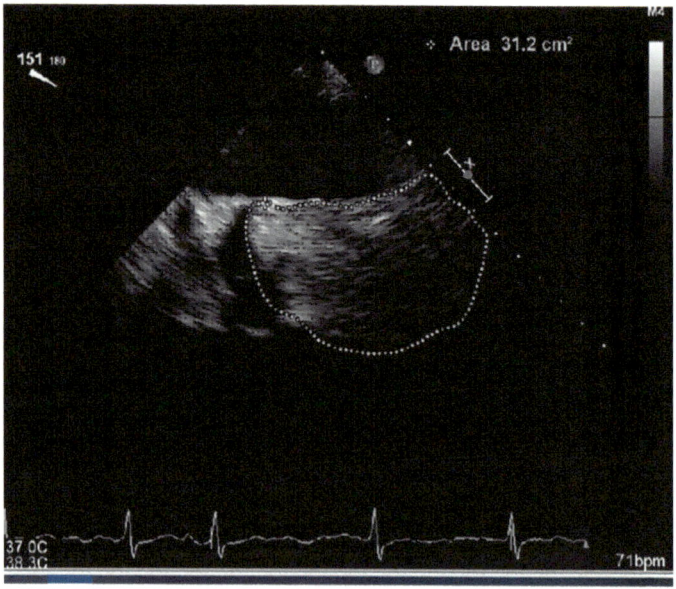

FIGURE 25.2 TEE bi-caval view, shows mass in RA

Follow up echocardiogram has not demonstrated any change in the size of RA masses. Then patient had coronary angiogram which revealed essentially normal coronary arteries.

She underwent open-heart surgery and resection of right atrial masses, reconstruction of left and right atrium and reconstruction of right superior pulmonary vein. Both tumors reported as benign lipomatous hypertrophy of inter atrial septum. Her post-op coarse complicated by presence of junctional rhythm, (SA nodal artery was divided during her surgery) and few episodes of atrial fibrillation.

She remained in junctional rhythm with no symptoms.

Her breast cancer was in remission and currently patient is treated by antihormone therapy.

Clinical Pearls

- Dumbbell-shaped mass sparing the fossa ovalis is characteristic for lipomatous hypertrophy of septum [1, 2].
- Lipomatous hypertrophy of septum is seen more frequently in obese elderly female patients [3, 4].
- On fluorodeoxyglucose (FDG)-positron emission tomography (PET) increased uptake of FDG could differentiate lipomatous hypertrophy of septum from other tumors. However, large size of this mass, and possibility of vena caval obstruction in the context of breast cancer necessitates surgical removal [5].
- 75% of cardiac masses are benign tumors like as myxomas [6].
- Metastatic mass is mostly secondary to esophageal cancer, melanoma, lymphoma, leukemia, lung cancer, breast cancer, renal carcinoma, hepatocellular carcinoma, and thyroid cancer [7].
- Presence of pericardial effusion should raise the suspicion for malignant cardiac masses like as sarcoma.

References

1. Ak K, Isbir S, Kepez A, Turkoz K, Elci E, Arsan S. Large lipomatous hypertrophy of the interventricular septum. Tex Heart Inst J. 2014;41(2):231–3.
2. Heyer C, Kagel T, Lemburg S, Bauer T, Nicolas V. Lipomatous hypertrophy of the interatrial septum. Chest. 2003;124(6):2068–73.
3. Bielicki G, Lukaszewski M, Kosiorowska K, et al. Lipomatous hypertrophy of the atrial septum – a benign heart anomaly causing unexpected surgical problems: a case report. BMC Cardiovasc Disord. 2018;18:152.
4. Nadra I. Lipomatous hypertrophy of the ineratrial septum; a commonly misdiagnosed mass often leading to unnecessary cardiac surgery. Heart. 2004;90(12):66.
5. Fan CM, Fischman AJ, Kwek BH, Abbara S, Aquino SL. Lipomatous hypertrophy of the interatrial septum: increased uptake on FDG PET. AJR Am J Roentgenol. 2005;184(1):339–42. PMID: 15615998. https://doi.org/10.2214/ajr.184.1.01840339.
6. Gowda RM, Khan IA, Nair CK, Mehta NJ, Vasavada BC, Sacchi TJ. Cardiac papillary fibroelastoma: a comprehensive analysis of 725 cases. Am Heart J. 2003;146(3):404–10. PMID: 12947356. https://doi.org/10.1016/S0002-8703(03)00249-7.
7. Reynen K, Köckeritz U, Strasser RH. Metastases to the heart. Ann Oncol. 2004;15(3):375–81. PMID: 14998838. https://doi.org/10.1093/annonc/mdh086.

Index

© The Author(s), under exclusive license to Springer Nature Switzerland AG 2021
A. Rohani, *Clinical Cases in Cardio-Oncology*, Clinical Cases in Cardiology, https://doi.org/10.1007/978-3-030-71155-9